T0258189

# GETTING RISK RIGHT

# GETTING RISK RIGHT
## Understanding the Science
## of Elusive Health Risks

GEOFFREY C. KABAT

COLUMBIA UNIVERSITY PRESS  NEW YORK

Columbia University Press
*Publishers Since 1893*
New York    Chichester, West Sussex
cup.columbia.edu
Copyright © 2017 Columbia University Press
All rights reserved

Library of Congress Cataloging-in-Publication Data
Names: Kabat, Geoffrey C., author.
Title: Getting risk right : understanding the science of elusive health risks /
Geoffrey C. Kabat.
Description: New York : Columbia University Press, [2017] |
Includes bibliographical references and index.
Identifiers: LCCN 2016008208 (print) | LCCN 2016008811 (ebook) |
ISBN 9780231166461 (cloth : alk. paper) | ISBN 9780231542852 (electronic)
Subjects: | MESH: Attitude to Health | Risk Assessment | Negativism |
Risk Factors | Environmental Exposure—adverse effects |
Health Education—methods
Classification: LCC RA776.5 (print) | LCC RA776.5 (ebook) |
NLM W 85 | DDC 613—dc23
LC record available at http://lccn.loc.gov/2016008208

Columbia University Press books are printed on permanent
and durable acid-free paper.
Printed in the United States of America

Cover design: Noah Arlow

*To the friends and colleagues who have
accompanied me on this journey*

*The first principle is that you must not fool yourself, and you are the easiest person to fool.*

—Richard Feynman

*What I am saying is that, in numerous areas that we call science, we have come to like our habitual ways, and our studies that can be continued indefinitely. We measure, we define, we compute, we analyze, but we do not exclude. And this is not the way to use our minds most effectively or to make the fastest progress in solving scientific questions.*

—John Platt

# CONTENTS

List of Illustrations    xi

Preface: Why Do Things That Are Unlikely to
Harm Us Get the Most Attention?    xiii

List of Abbreviations    xxi

1   THE ILLUSION OF VALIDITY AND
THE POWER OF "NEGATIVE THINKING"    1

2   SPLENDORS AND MISERIES OF ASSOCIATIONS    8

3   WHEN RISK GOES VIRAL: Biases and Bandwagons    32

4   DO CELL PHONES CAUSE BRAIN CANCER?
A Tale of Two Sciences    59

5   HORMONAL CONFUSION: The Contested
Science of Endocrine Disruption    85

6   DEADLY REMEDY: A Mysterious Disease, a Medicinal Herb, and the Recognition of a Worldwide Public Health Threat      116

7   HPV, CANCER, AND BEYOND: The Anatomy of a Triumph      144

CONCLUSION      175

Appendix: List of Interviews      181

Notes      183

Glossary      209

Bibliography      221

Index      237

# ILLUSTRATIONS

Figure 2.1   Association between an exposure and a disease.   15

Figure 2.2   Any association we study is embedded in a thicket of other correlations.   16

Figure 2.3   "Correlation globe" showing correlations among environmental pollutants and clinical variables.   17

Figure 2.4   "Today's Random Medical News"   21

Figure 3.1   Interactions between scientific findings and the different communities that use them.   33

Figure 3.2   "When your only tool is a trebuchet, every problem looks like a siege."   42

Figure 4.1   The electromagnetic spectrum.   62

Figure 4.2   Number of wireless subscribers and brain cancer incidence in the United States, 1977–2012.   77

Figure 5.1   Chemical structures of several compounds with differing estrogenic potencies.   92

Figure 6.1   Map showing distribution of Balkan endemic nephropathy regions.   123

Figure 7.1   Map of subequatorial Africa showing areas with Burkitt's lymphoma.   146

Figure 7.2   Cervical cancer mortality by country.   163

Figure 7.3   HPV DNA prevalence in different regions of the world.   164

Figure 7.4   Phylogenetic tree showing 170 HPV types.   168

# PREFACE

## WHY DO THINGS THAT ARE UNLIKELY TO HARM US GET THE MOST ATTENTION?

The modern world, the advanced technological world in which we live, is a dangerous place. Or, at least, that is the message that, with metronomic regularity, seems to jump out at us at every turn. The news media bombard us with reports of the latest threat to our health lurking in our food, air, water, and the environment, and these messages are often reinforced by regulatory agencies, activist groups, and scientists themselves. In recent years we have been encouraged to worry about deadly toxins in baby bottles, food, and cosmetics; carcinogenic radiation from power lines and cell phones; and harm from vaccines and genetically modified foods, to name just a few of the more prominent scares.

When looked at even the least bit critically, many of the scares that get high-profile attention turn out to be based on weak or erroneous findings that were hardly ready for prime time. Consider two recent reports that came out a few days apart. One proclaimed that ingesting the chemical BPA in the minute quantities normally encountered in daily life may increase fat deposition in the body.[1] The second suggested that babies born to mothers living in proximity to sites where hydraulic fracturing, or "fracking," is being used to extract natural gas from rock formations may have reduced birth weight.[2] Reports like these have a visceral impact. They inform us that a new and hitherto unsuspected threat has taken up residence in our immediate environment, in our body, or in the bodies of people like us. The impact is similar to coming home and sensing that there is a malevolent intruder in your home.

In the two instances cited above, a quick look at the original studies on which these news items were based would have revealed the crucial point: there are a large number of substantial leaps—over many intervening steps or linkages—between the putative cause and the putative effect. At each point in the logical chain of causation there is the opportunity for unwarranted assumptions, poor measurement, ignoring crucial factors, and other methodological problems to enter in. Any erroneous link would invalidate the overall linkage that the article is positing and that the news reports trumpet. But, by a mysterious cognitive process, we tend to block out these considerations and accept the validity of what is a tenuous connection that would need extensive buttressing to be worthy of concern. The process of questioning how seriously such results should be taken is an effortful, rational process that cannot compete with the visceral impact of the alert telling us that we are under threat. Even those who are in a position to know better can be unsettled by reports like these.

Our response to such reports is often influenced by another cognitive process that we are usually unaware of. Independent of how solid the underlying science is, the new result may *sound true* to our ears because it appears to fit in with a broader theme or narrative, which is beyond dispute. Thus any report alleging effects of exposure to environmental pollution may gain plausibility from the incontestable fact that we humans are having a profound and unprecedented impact on the global environment. But, in spite of what seems true, the results of any study need to be evaluated critically, and in the light of other evidence, to see if they stand up. One cannot judge a scientific finding based on whether it conforms to our expectations.

The visceral impact of these scares helps explain how, in different instances, the scientific and regulatory communities, various activist groups, self-appointed health gurus, and the media could all get involved and make their contribution to giving these and similar questionable findings currency.

Although news reports of these threats always make reference to the latest scientific study or measurement, the scares that erupt into the public consciousness often have only a tenuous connection to hard scientific evidence or logic. Many people sense this intuitively, since a report pointing to a hazard is often followed closely by another finding no evidence of a hazard, or even finding a benefit from the supposed nemesis. Furthermore, they sense that people aren't dropping like flies from the numerous dangers alleged to permeate modern life. Certainly the periodic reports raising the terrifying possibility that using a cell phone could cause brain cancer have done nothing to slow the unparalleled spread of this technology. And yet this omnipresent noise and the continual procession of new threats to our health take their toll and have real consequences, although these get little attention from those who so vigorously promote the existence of a hazard.

\* \* \*

Information about what factors truly have an important impact on health is a vital commodity that has the potential to affect lives, but the succession of health scares creates a fog that confuses people about what they should pay attention to. People paralyzed, or merely distracted, by the latest imaginary threat may become desensitized to health messages and be less likely to pay attention to things that matter and that are actually within their control—like stopping smoking, controlling their weight, having their children vaccinated, and going for effective screening. Concerning the cell phone scare, in 2008 Otis Brawley, chief medical officer for the American Cancer Society, commented, "I am afraid that if we pull the fire alarm, scaring people unnecessarily, and actually diverting their attention from things that they should be doing, then when we do pull the fire alarm for a public health emergency, we won't have the credibility for them to listen to us."[3]

In addition, the exaggeration and distortion of health risks can lead to the formulation of well-intended but wrongheaded policies that can actually do harm. Perhaps the best example of this is the overzealous focus on the presumed benefits of a low-fat diet in the 1990s. Both the federal government and the public health community embraced this doctrine, and the food industry complied by reducing the fat content of a wide range of processed foods. However, something needed to be substituted for the missing fat, and sugar filled this role. This large-scale and dramatic change—sometimes referred to as the "SnackWell phenomenon"—has been credited with making a substantial contribution to increasing rates of obesity.[4]

There is also a cost in missed opportunities. We need to recalibrate our judgment as to what is a problem, since, if resources are spent to remediate a trivial or nonexistent hazard, clearly fewer resources will be available to devote to more promising work that may turn out to have major benefits. This is especially critical since, as the outbreaks of SARS, avian flu, Ebola, and now Zika virus make clear, new and serious threats to public health will continue to arise.

Finally, the confusion caused by conflicting scientific findings, polarizing controversies, and wrongheaded policies erodes the public's trust in science and in institutions mandated to promote research and apply its results to improving public health. In fact, in spite of the unprecedented progress in many fields of science over the past sixty years, the public's trust in science has declined since the decades immediately following the Second World War.[5]

* * *

Although we are dependent on science and medicine as never before, there is widespread confusion among nonscientists about how to make sense of the flood of information that is being produced at an ever-increasing rate regarding factors that influence health. A recent survey by the American Institute for Cancer Research (AICR) found that "awareness of key cancer risk factors was alarmingly low, while more Americans than ever cling to unproven links."[6] The survey results showed that fewer than half of Americans know the real risks, whereas high percentages of respondents worry about risks for which there is little persuasive support. The latter include pesticide residues on produce, food additives, genetically modified foods, stress, and hormones in beef.

If the AICR report is correct, it is worth asking how such a situation arose in the first place and what factors perpetuate it. Scientists who are in a position to know, including epidemiologists who have devoted their careers to evaluating health risks, have expressed their frustration—at times verging on despair—at this state of affairs. And those who have given thought to the problem acknowledge that their work makes no small contribution to the confusion.[7]

More generally, it is widely recognized that there is a crisis in the field of biomedicine, characterized by a "culture of hyper-competitiveness." In this environment, scientists may feel the need to overstate the importance of their work in order to attract attention and obtain funding. Other symptoms of this climate are a "lack of transparent reporting of results" and an increasing frequency of published results that cannot be replicated.[8]

So how is it possible for a nonscientist to distinguish between what deserves serious attention and what is questionable in the torrent of conflicting scientific findings and health recommendations? What is needed above all is to develop an understanding of what solid and important findings look like and how they are established, as well as developing a healthy skepticism toward results that may be tenuous but get amplified because they speak to our deepest fears.

Sorting out what is known on questions relating to health and interpreting the evidence critically is a challenging task, since different groups of scientists can interpret the same results differently and can emphasize different findings. When the evidence is weak or conflicting, as it often is, subjective judgment assumes a more important role, and scientists, being human, are not immune to their own biases.

When it comes to communicating research results to the public, there is an enormous gulf separating the scientific community from the general public. The scientific literature presupposes a familiarity with the subject matter, concepts, terminology, and methods, knowledge that is acquired only through a long apprenticeship. Even the most basic terms, such as *risk, hazard, association, exposure, environment*, and *bias*, mean one thing to the specialist and often have a very different meaning in general usage. The very way of thinking about a particular question can differ radically between the specialist and the public. In addition to the challenge of communicating inherently technical results, findings about factors that may affect our health have a strong emotional resonance that does not pertain to other scientific questions, such as the nature of "dark matter," the origins of life, or the nature of consciousness.

If knowledge about what affects our health is an invaluable commodity, dispelling the mystery and confusion surrounding the science in this area could not be a more urgent task. A number of recent books have sought to explain the power of belief and the increasing prevalence of "denialism," that is, the holding of beliefs that conflict with well-established science. From a variety of perspectives—journalistic, psychological, sociological, and political—their authors have attempted to shed light on the processes that shape and reinforce erroneous beliefs.[9] Other books have done an excellent job of explaining how epidemiology and clinical medicine enable the discovery of new and important knowledge.[10] However, little attention has been devoted to the challenges confronting research in the area of health risks and the ways in which biases and agendas endemic to scientific research, as well as tendencies operating in the wider society, can affect how findings are communicated to the public. Only by examining the interactions between scientists and the different groups and institutions that make use of research findings can we begin to make sense of the successes and failures of the science that addresses health risks.

In an earlier book I examined a number of alleged health hazards that received an enormous amount of attention and generated widespread anxiety.[11] As an epidemiologist doing primary research on some of these questions, I could see that the public perception of these issues was badly skewed and distorted. When examined in a dispassionate way, these high-profile risks turned out to be much less important than was claimed. But the studies that got reported in the media and acted on by scientific and regulatory panels were "scientific" studies. So I wanted to explore how this could happen, and what factors contributed to the inflation of these health risks. Where did the process go wrong?

The short answer is that when scientific research focuses on a potential hazard that may affect the population at large, researchers themselves, regulatory agencies, advocacy groups, and journalists reporting on the story tend to emphasize what appear to be positive findings, even when the results are inconsistent, the risks may be small in magnitude and uncertain, and other, more important factors may be ignored.

In examining these inflated risks, I was struck by a paradox. In contrast to questions that provoke needless alarm but which can persist for a long time without any resolution or progress, we hear little about other stories that represent extraordinary triumphs of science at its best.

The present book asks the question, what does successful scientific research in the area of health and health risks look like, and how does it differ from the research that draws our attention to sensational but poorly supported or ambiguous findings that never seem to get confirmed but have great potential to inspire fear? By examining examples of these contrasting outcomes of scientific research, I hope to show how the scientific enterprise, at its best, can succeed in elucidating difficult questions, while other issues that attract a great deal of attention may yield little in the way of important new knowledge.

\* \* \*

During work on this book, I have benefited from discussions with a number of colleagues and friends. Several colleagues answered my questions—often repeated waves of questions and follow-up questions—in interviews conducted in person or via e-mail. Some of these colleagues and friends read chapters of the manuscript and offered corrections, suggestions, and encouragement. I especially want to thank Robert Tarone, David Parmacek, Daniel Doerge, Anders Ahlbom, Robert Burk, Mark Schiffman, Richard Sharpe, Arthur Grollman, Robert Adair, Lawrence Silbart, Kamal Chaouachi, David Savitz, Gio Gori, Daniel Kabat, Steven Stellman, John Moulder, Allen Wilcox, and John Ioannidis. From the beginning, my editor at Columbia University Press, Patrick Fitzgerald, has been enthusiastic and excited about the project. Bridget Flannery-McCoy of the Press gave me valuable comments on an early draft, and Ryan Groendyk, Lisa Hamm, and Anita O'Brien did an expert job of shepherding the manuscript through the publication process. As always, my wife, Roberta Kabat, has been a consistent source of clear-eyed judgment, critical intelligence, and unflagging moral support.

# ABBREVIATIONS

| | |
|---|---|
| AAN | aristolochic acid nephropathy |
| AICR | American Institute for Cancer Research |
| BEN | Balkan endemic nephropathy |
| BMJ | British Medical Journal |
| BPA | bisphenol A |
| CAM | complementary and alternative medicine |
| CDC | Centers for Disease Control and Prevention |
| CHN | Chinese herbs nephropathy |
| CIN | cervical intraepithelial neoplasia |
| CTIA | Cellular Communications Industry Association |
| DDE | dichlorodiphenyldichloroethylene |
| DES | diethylstilbestrol |
| DDT | dichlorodiphenyltrichloroethane |
| DMAA | 1,3-dimethylamylamine |
| DSHEA | Dietary Supplement Health and Education Act |
| EBV | Epstein-Barr virus |
| EC | European Commission |
| ED | endocrine disruption |
| EDC | endocrine disrupting chemicals |
| EFSA | European Food Safety Authority |
| EHP | *Environmental Health Perspectives* |
| EMF | electromagnetic field |

| | |
|---|---|
| EPA | Environmental Protection Agency |
| FCC | Federal Communications Commission |
| FDA | Food and Drug Administration |
| GMOs | genetically modified organisms |
| HBV | hepatitis B virus |
| HPV | human papillomavirus |
| HSV | herpes simplex virus |
| IARC | International Agency for Research on Cancer |
| ICNIRP | International Commission on Non-Ionizing Radiation Protection |
| JNCI | *Journal of the National Cancer Institute* |
| MMR | measles, mumps, and rubella |
| NCI | National Cancer Institute |
| NCS | National Children's Study |
| NIEHS | National Institute of Environmental Health Sciences |
| OR | odds ratio |
| p53 | tumor suppressor gene p53 |
| PCBs | polychlorinated biphenyls |
| PCR | polymerase chain reaction |
| PLoS | *Public Library of Science* |
| PNAS | *Proceedings of the National Academy of Sciences* |
| PV | papillomavirus |
| RF | radiofrequency energy |
| SAR | specific absorption rate |
| SCENIHR | Scientific Committee on Emerging and Newly Identified Health Risks |
| TCDD | 2,3,7,8-tetrachlorodibenzodioxin (dioxin) |
| TDS | testicular dysgenesis syndrome |
| VLP | virus-like particle |
| WHO | World Health Organization |

# GETTING RISK RIGHT

# 1

# The Illusion of Validity and the Power of "Negative Thinking"

It is the peculiar and perpetual error of the human understanding to be more moved and excited by affirmatives than by negatives.

The root of all superstition is that men observe when things hit but not when they miss; and commit to memory the one and forget and pass over the other.

—FRANCIS BACON

During World War II the Allies carried out a strategic bombing campaign against the German industrial heartland from airfields in Britain. The main workhorse of the campaign was the Lancaster four-engine bomber, which, owing to its weight and slow speed, suffered punishing losses from German night fighters. By one estimate, the chances of a crew reaching the end of a thirty-mission tour were about 25 percent. The British military called in experts, including the young Freeman Dyson, to determine how to reduce the staggering casualty rates. Owing to their heavy armor plating and gun turrets, the planes were forced to fly at a low altitude and were painted black to make them less visible during their night runs. Dyson tells of a vice air marshal, Sir Ralph Cochrane, who proposed ripping out the gun turrets and other dead weight from one of the Lancasters, painting it white, and flying it high over Germany. But the military command rejected this audacious experiment owing to what Dyson, following Daniel Kahneman, calls the "illusion of validity"—the deep-seated human need to believe that our actions are well-founded.[1]

All those involved in the air war believed in the tightly knit bomber crew, with the gunner playing a crucial role in defending the aircraft, and the pilot using his experience to take evasive actions. Dyson writes, "The illusion that experience would help them to survive was essential to their morale. After all, they could see in every squadron a few revered and experienced old-timer crews who had completed one tour and had volunteered to return for a second tour. It was obvious to everyone that the old-timers survived because they were more skillful. Nobody wanted to believe that the old-timers survived only because they were more lucky."

When Dyson undertook a careful analysis of the correlation between the experience of the crews and their loss rates, taking into account the possible distorting effects of weather and geography, he found that experience had no effect on whether a plane returned home. "So far as I could tell, whether a crew lived or died was purely a matter of chance. Their belief in the life-saving effect of experience was an illusion."

Dyson's demonstration that experience had no effect on losses should have provided strong support for Cochrane's idea of tearing out the gun turrets. But it did nothing of the sort. He tells us that "everyone at Bomber Command, from the commander in chief to the flying crews, continued to believe in the illusion. The crews continued to die, experienced and inexperienced alike, until Germany was overrun and the war was finally ended."

It took another outsider to come up with a dazzling insight into the reasons for the heavy toll on British bombers. Abraham Wald was a Jewish mathematician from Eastern Europe who had come to the United States in the late 1930s to escape persecution. During the war he used his knowledge of statistics to analyze the problem of the aircraft losses. Analysts had proposed adding armor to those areas of the aircraft that showed the most damage. What Wald realized was that the damage sustained by the aircraft that returned safely represented areas that were not fatal to the plane's survival. The fact that there were areas of the returning planes that showed no damage led him to surmise that these were the vulnerable spots that must have led to the loss of the planes to enemy fire. Thus it was these areas that needed to be reinforced.[2]

Making an inspired leap, Wald posited that there must be a crucial difference in the pattern of damage between those bombers that returned and those that did not. He saw that the missing data—the bombers that never made it back—provided the key to the problem, and he analyzed the pattern of *nonfatal* damage displayed by the returning bombers to intuit the pattern of fatal damage to the planes that did not return. What his analysis showed was that the planes' engines were vulnerable and needed shielding.

Wald's approach to estimating aircraft survivability was used during World War II, as well as by the U.S. Navy and Air Force during the Korean and Vietnam Wars. Today his analysis—which was carried out without computers—is considered a seminal contribution to statistics and specifically to the problem of "missing data." Writing about Wald's work on aircraft survivability in the leading statistics journal in 1984, two statisticians concluded that, "while the field of statistics has grown considerably since the early 1940's, Wald's work on this problem is difficult to improve upon. . . . By the sheer power of his intuition, [he] was . . . able to deal with both structural and inferential questions in a definitive way."[3]

More broadly, Wald's analysis provides an example of how crucial it is to consider the full range of relevant data, rather than confining oneself to a biased sample (i.e., the planes that returned safely) or to the usual categories. It is an inspired example of what we refer to (perhaps too lazily) today as "thinking outside the box." It underscores the need to be open to new ways of seeing, going beyond the limits of our habitual thinking, and looking for answers in places where we might not immediately think to look.[4]

In fact, Dyson's "illusion of validity" and Wald's "negative thinking" represent two sides of a single coin. Taken together, the stories of Dyson and Wald provide inspired examples of overcoming the impediments to thinking afresh about a problem, divesting oneself of preconceptions and habitual ways of looking at things. We all tend to focus on certain salient aspects of a problem, and these can obscure other aspects, which may be essential to consider. Experts are not exempt from this tendency, which, it has been noted, is particularly in evidence among those who formulate policy.[5]

\* \* \*

Since World War II, science has made remarkable progress in medicine, genetics, molecular biology, and epidemiology. And yet, in spite of this progress, our understanding of what causes many chronic diseases and how to prevent them is still humblingly limited. Furthermore, widespread confusion reigns about what are the real threats that are likely to affect our lives. For example, there are controversies raging within the scientific community or wider society regarding a wide range of issues, including radiofrequency radiation from cellular telephones and other wireless technology, "endocrine disrupting chemicals" including pesticides and other contaminants in our food and consumer products, what constitutes a healthy diet, vaccines, obesity, genetically modified foods, the use of hydraulic fracturing ("fracking") to extract oil and gas, alternative and complementary medicine, and particulate air pollution—to name some of the more prominent topics.

These threats, which are so much in view, tap into reflexes that allowed our ancestors to survive hundreds of thousands of years ago in the African savannah. But the instinctual reaction that served us well when the task of not being eaten by a predator was paramount is less suited to the modern world, which is a much more complicated environment to navigate. It is not that we are wrong to be mistrustful and wary of our environment or to question information put out by the authorities, but when we adopt an extreme position—embracing conspiracy theories and rejecting objective evidence that comes from impartial sources—we are apt to fall for the "illusion of validity" and fail to recognize other real dangers.

Similarly, when scientists become wedded to a particular hypothesis and resist considering contradictory evidence and alternative explanations, they narrow their field of vision and close off what may be more productive lines of inquiry.

This brings us to the two very different outcomes of scientific research in the area of health and health risks that are the focus of this book. At the outset, it needs to be said that the vast majority of research never attracts the attention of the media or the public. So the contrast I am setting up is one of extremes.

Research that succeeds in uncovering new knowledge involves the painstaking process of formulating a hypothesis, obtaining meaningful data, ruling out artifacts and overcoming biases, comparing results from different research groups, and considering and excluding alternative explanations at each step of the way. At the heart of this process is a tension between the researcher's hypothesis and the evolving evidence bearing on it. It is only natural that a researcher can become deeply invested in a particular hypothesis. But, at the same time, he or she has to be the most relentless critic of the hypothesis and be willing to modify or reject it if it conflicts with the evidence. In pursuing an initial idea, a researcher will often be led to a more promising idea that was not envisaged at the outset. All this takes place out of the spotlight, for the simple reason that until one has followed the line of inquiry and obtained a solid result, there is no reason to get the media and the public stirred up about the possible significance of the work. (An added motivation for caution is that one doesn't want to end up looking like a fool.)

Some hypotheses may be weak but may nevertheless merit study. If research does not provide support for the hypothesis, in due course it would normally be abandoned for other lines of research. However, in cases where a weak hypothesis touches on a topic that has the potential to galvanize public concern, what is at heart a scientific question can attract the attention of nonscientists, including regulators, funding agencies, advocates, journalists, and others. When such an issue is framed in a narrow way—is X a problem?—a way that restricts attention to the putative threat and fails to put it in perspective, it can take on a life of its own. Regulators may feel the need to consider the question. Funding agencies may decide to support further research. These actions, which attract news coverage and generate more concern in the public, keep the issue in the public eye. Some scientists may believe that there is evidence to support the hypothesis and may have a strong stake in it. Furthermore, because their findings speak to deep-seated fears relating to a publicized issue, the work of these scientists can be championed by advocates who believe that they are telling the truth, in opposition to "establishment scientists," who are minimizing or suppressing a real problem. We will see examples of this second outcome of research in the stories of cell phones, endocrine-disrupting chemicals, and particularly BPA.

\* \* \*

It is a striking paradox that the stories concerning the causes of chronic disease that get the most attention often involve findings that are questionable but that have the power to arouse anxiety, whereas stories involving painstaking, incremental work that, over time, leads to major, life-saving advances get little attention. Both types of stories are the product of "science," and yet, depending on the research question and the social context surrounding that question, the prospects for uncovering new and important knowledge can be radically different. Strong scientific results speak for themselves—they lead to tangible and reproducible results. In contrast, when research fails to make solid progress in an area that arouses public concern, it is only too easy for researchers and advocates to offer up weak or erroneous results to the public as meaningful findings. Research that for various reasons goes off the rails and ends up misleading us rather than yielding useful knowledge has been variously referred to as "bad science," "voodoo science," "cargo cult science," "pathological science," and "parascience."[6] Successful research exists in a separate realm, and there are many valuable accounts of the process of scientific discovery.[7] However, rarely have the two very different outcomes been forced to confront each other. What follows is an exploration of what distinguishes these two contrasting outcomes of scientific research.

Chapter 2 describes the fundamentals of observational studies in the area of public health. Studies reporting associations between an exposure and a disease vary greatly in import depending on prior knowledge regarding the association, the ability to measure the exposure and the disease condition accurately, and other methodological factors. Thus it is essential to realize that not all reported associations are created equal. However, because it is challenging to identify the important causes of complex chronic diseases that are multiply determined and that may take decades to develop, there is a tendency to latch onto findings that appear to point to a cause, even when the methodology is weak. If science in this area means anything, it means the uncompromisingly critical assessment of the relevant evidence on a question.

Chapter 3 describes how science in this area is embedded in a society that is highly attuned to the latest potential threat or breakthrough. Findings from rudimentary studies often are reported as if they were likely to be true when, in fact, most research findings are false or exaggerated, and the more dramatic the result, the less likely it is to be true. The public's hunger for novel information about health threats and breakthroughs creates a fertile soil for biases that come into play in interpreting the results of observational studies and disseminating findings to the public. Reports of exaggerated findings can, in turn, give rise to "information cascades"— highly publicized campaigns that can sow needless alarm and lead to misguided regulation and policies.

The question of whether exposure to radiofrequency energy (RF) causes brain cancer arose over twenty years ago and is still a cause of controversy and confusion. Chapter 4 examines what science has to say about the disturbing possibility that the worldwide adoption of a novel technology within a short time span could be causing a terrifying fatal disease. In fact, extensive research carried out over two decades provides no strong or consistent evidence to support this possibility.

Chapter 5 explores the main lines of the preoccupation with "endocrine disrupting chemicals" in the environment; how this question first arose; what we have learned from decades of research, including false ideas based on poor data that got enormous attention; and how to make sense of a bitter controversy that is currently raging in the scientific and regulatory communities in Europe and the United States.

Chapter 6 describes a little-known story linking a long-standing, enigmatic disease in the Balkans to dietary exposure to a toxic herb that has been used in traditional cultures throughout history, right up to the present. The mystery was fortuitously illuminated by a dramatic outbreak of kidney disease among women attending a weight-loss clinic in Brussels. Research on the potent toxin and carcinogen aristolochic acid contained in certain varieties of the herb *Aristolochia* has led to new insights into the carcinogenic process, as well as highlighting the threat to public health posed by the woefully inadequate regulation of thousands of products marketed as "dietary supplements."

Chapter 7 recounts how the long-standing question of what causes cervical cancer led, over a period of thirty years, to the identification of a small number of highly specific carcinogenic subtypes of the human papillomavirus (HPV) and to the understanding that persistent infection with one or more of these subtypes is necessary to cause the disease. This knowledge in turn has led to the development of vaccines that have the potential to virtually eliminate cervical cancer—a major cause of cancer death among women worldwide—as well as to fundamental new knowledge about how the virus evolved to cause cancer.

The conclusion emphasizes the need for a more nuanced and realistic view of science, which acknowledges the enormous challenges, promotes skepticism toward widely circulated but questionable ideas, and at the same time pays attention to what science can achieve at its best.

# 2

# Splendors and Miseries of Associations

The apparent endemicity of bad research behavior is alarming.
In their quest for telling a compelling story, scientists too often sculpt
their data to fit their preferred theory of the world.

—RICHARD HORTON

## EBOLA AND BPA

In October 2014 a paper appeared in a leading scientific journal purporting to show that volunteers who handled cash register receipts after using a hand sanitizer absorbed enough of the chemical bisphenol A, or BPA, from the thermal paper to put them at increased risk of a number of serious diseases.[1] This was only the latest in a long line of scientific studies linking BPA, which is widely used to line food containers and certain plastic bottles, to a wide range of adverse health effects. In fact, both the specific findings and the interpretation were in conflict with extensive evidence from high-quality scientific studies as well as reports by various national and international agencies that argued against the existence of a hazard. Yet the authors of the paper claimed that they were picking up a true phenomenon that other scientists were missing, due either to faulty methodology or to conflicts of interest and subservience to industry.

There is nothing unusual about the paper. Rather, it is representative of a genre that has become increasingly common in the health sciences literature, particularly where researchers study the potential contribution of environmental exposures to the risk of developing serious disease. However, the paper happened to come out at a time when the Ebola epidemic in West Africa was continuing to outstrip massive efforts to bring it under control. It is instructive to compare the putative hazards stemming from this most modern of technologies (thermal printing paper) and the all-too-real threat posed by the virus that originated in an isolated and remote region of Central Africa.

In the first case, we have an exposure that is habitually described as "ubiquitous." Virtually everyone is exposed to cash register receipts, some of which contain BPA, which is used as a developer. Additionally, it is a widely publicized fact that many synthetic chemicals, like BPA, can be detected in the urine of most people, including children, in developed countries. These are the operative facts, and often they are enough to trigger concern. What few people who are concerned about BPA realize is that the levels of the chemical that are absorbed from food containers (the major source) are miniscule. Furthermore, the chemical is almost totally (>99%) metabolized and excreted in the urine, even in infants, and therefore does not accumulate in the body. Is it possible that exposure to BPA poses some hazard to some people? Yes, we can never rule out the possibility of some effect. But based on a large amount of accumulated scientific evidence, any adverse effect, if one exists, is likely to be very small. In other words, we can't say that an adverse effect is impossible, but we can say that it is implausible.

If a connection between exposure to BPA and human health is tenuous and lacking any strong scientific support, the effects of the Ebola virus were all too real, immediate, and horrible. Daily images and news reports from West Africa conveyed the stark and unmistakable reality: people stricken by the virus lying in the street, dying where they collapsed, with bystanders looking on helplessly; workers encased in "moon suits" spraying chlorine disinfectant in the tracks of patients being led to a clinic. The connection between the exposure and its effects could not be clearer. The virus is spread only by direct contact with the body fluids of those with symptoms, but such contact is highly infectious—so infectious that health care workers carefully removing their protective clothing could inadvertently become infected. In those who were infected, the mortality rate was roughly 60 percent. By the time the World Health Organization declared the outbreak over in 2016 there were 28,637 known cases and 11,315 deaths.

So BPA and Ebola can be taken to represent two very different types of "health risks"—two extremes—one, theoretical and likely to be undetectable; the other, all too real. Their juxtaposition raises fundamental questions about how risks are perceived and acted on, and what aspects are most salient and receive attention and what aspects are ignored. To Americans, the drama unfolding in West Africa—one of the top news stories of 2014—appeared almost surreal owing to the vast socioeconomic and cultural distance separating us from these societies. More than anything, the images conjured up the alien and nightmarish logic of movies like *Outbreak* and *Contagion*. However, it took only one infected traveler from Liberia to present at a Dallas hospital with a fever for Ebola to take on a drastically different meaning. The hospital staff, which had no prior experience treating the disease, was caught off guard and did not initially consider Ebola. By the time the disease was recognized it was too late, and the patient had died. One of the treating nurses, however, was infected with the virus and was transferred to the National Institutes of Health, where she recovered. These events were enough to send the country into a paroxysm of fear regarding Ebola. One survey estimated that 40 percent of Americans were concerned that a large outbreak of the disease would occur in the United States within the next year.[2]

What is most striking about the response to the handful of Ebola cases in the United States is how certain facts registered, whereas others of equal or greater importance were lost sight of. What accounts for the terrible toll of Ebola in West Africa is the woefully inadequate infrastructure and medical resources in countries that are among the poorest in the world. In addition, early on in the outbreak, people did not trust their government's information campaigns regarding the disease and were reluctant to follow its directives. If infected people are identified early and adequate treatment is available, the odds of survival are greatly improved. In the United States, with a high level of medical care and with screening of passengers coming from Africa, the chances of Ebola becoming a serious problem were very slight. In contrast, the seasonal flu spreads easily through the air by means of exhaled droplets and is responsible for tens of thousands of deaths each year, mainly in the very young and the elderly. But few Americans worry about dying from seasonal flu.

I have focused on the contrast between these two health threats—BPA and Ebola—for two reasons. First, they represent two extremes of "risk." In the case of Ebola, the risk is so immediate and potent that no study is needed to demonstrate causality. In the case of BPA, if a risk exists at all, it is a great many orders of magnitude more subtle. Second, the contrast between Ebola and BPA highlights the widespread and dangerous confusion that surrounds both real and potential health risks.

\* \* \*

We are awash in reports, discussions, and controversies regarding a long list of exposures that, we are told, may affect our health: genetically modified

(GM) foods; "endocrine disrupting chemicals" in the environment; cell phones and their base stations; electromagnetic fields from power lines and electrical appliances; pesticides and herbicides currently in use, such as atrazine, neonicotinoids, and glyphosate, or those used in the past, such as DDT; fine particle air pollution; electronic cigarettes; smokeless tobacco; excess weight and obesity; vaccines; alcohol; salt intake; red and processed meat; screening for cancer; and dietary and herbal supplements. Each of these issues is distinct and needs to be assessed on its own terms. Each has a body of scientific literature devoted to it. Yet on many of these questions there are sharply conflicting views. In some cases (e.g., endocrine disrupting chemicals, pesticides, salt intake, smokeless tobacco products, and electronic cigarettes), this stems from splits within the scientific community, which are mirrored in the wider society. In other cases (GM foods, vaccines), there may be an overwhelming consensus among scientists against something being a risk, but vocal advocates espousing contrary views can have a strong influence on susceptible members of the public. It should be noted that in some cases, the public's persisting belief in a hazard that is no longer supported by the scientific community has its origin either in scientific uncertainty (GM foods) or in work that was later shown to be fraudulent (vaccines).[3] In this welter of discordant scientific findings and competing claims, how are we to make sense of what is important and what is well-founded?

Understanding the sources of confusion and error surrounding the steady stream of findings from scientific studies is not just an academic concern. Beliefs about what constitutes a health threat have real consequences and affect lives, as four current issues demonstrate:

- An outbreak of measles affecting 149 people in eight U.S. states and Canada and Mexico in the winter of 2014–15 has been traced to Disneyland in California. That outbreak has been attributed to the failure of parents to allow their children to be vaccinated, based on unfounded health concerns or due to religious beliefs.[4]
- With forty million smokers in the United States, many of whom want to quit, the resistance on the part of many in the public health community to acknowledge the enormous benefits of electronic cigarettes and low-carcinogen, moist smokeless tobacco as alternatives to smoking represents an abdication of reason.[5]
- Food-borne illnesses caused by Salmonella, E. coli, and several other pathogens are responsible for at least 30,000 deaths each year in the United States.[6]

• The powerful health supplements industry, abetted by inadequate government regulation and safeguards, markets products of unknown purity and composition to adults and minors.[7] While the majority of these products may be harmless, there have been enough cases of organ damage and death that have been convincingly linked to specific products that the whole area of dietary supplements deserves attention. A recent report has estimated that 23,000 emergency room visits each year in the United States are due to adverse events involving dietary supplements.[8]

It is symptomatic of the state of the public discourse concerning health risks that issues like these do not have anywhere near the same salience as the typical scare-of-the-week.

To begin to make sense of the conflicting scientific findings and disputes bedeviling these questions, at the outset we need to be aware of the type of studies that are the source of many of these findings, and how they work. One doesn't have to take a course in epidemiology to understand the essentials of these studies, what they can achieve, and what their limitations are. It is simply that, in most journalistic reporting of results, for understandable reasons, the underlying assumptions and limitations are rarely even touched on. This is not too surprising in view of the fact that researchers themselves often fail to hedge their results with the needed qualifications. After a brief primer on how to think about epidemiologic studies, we can proceed to look at what is required to go from an initial finding regarding a possible link between an exposure and a disease to obtaining more solid evidence that this link is likely to represent cause and effect and to account for a significant proportion of disease. Many of the findings we hear about regarding certain questions are tentative and conflicting, and we need to distinguish between such findings and those where we have firm knowledge concerning risks that actually make a difference. This chapter addresses that crucial distinction.

## WHAT IS AN OBSERVATIONAL STUDY AND WHAT CAN IT TELL US?

Many of the findings concerning this or that factor that may affect our health stem from epidemiologic or "observational studies." The term *observational* is used in contrast to "experimental" studies, which are considered the "gold standard" in medical research but which, for ethical reasons, cannot be used to test the effects of harmful exposures in human beings. Observational studies of this kind involve the collecting of information on an exposure of interest in a defined population and relating this information to the occurrence of a disease of interest. Broadly speaking, two main types of study design are widely used. First, cases of a disease of interest can be identified in hospitals (or disease registries) and enrolled in a study, and a suitable comparison group ("controls") can be selected. This is referred to as a *case-control* study. Information is then obtained from cases and controls in order to identify factors that are associated with the occurrence of the disease. Note that in this type of study, cases have already developed the disease of interest, and information on past exposure is collected going back in time and usually depends on the subject's recall. The case-control design is particularly suited for the study of rare diseases. Owing to its retrospective nature, however, it is subject to "recall bias," since the information on exposure may be affected by the diagnosis, and cases may respond to questions about their past exposure differently from controls.

Using another approach, the researcher can identify a defined population—such as workers in a particular industry, members of a health plan, members of a specific profession, or volunteers enrolled by the American Cancer Society—and collect information on their health status and behaviors, as well as clinical specimens at the time of enrollment. The members of the "cohort" are then followed over time for the occurrence of disease and death. Information on exposure can then be related to the development of a disease of interest. This type of study is variously referred to as a *cohort*, *prospective*, or *longitudinal* study. Since, in this type of study, information on exposure is collected prior to the development of disease, the problem of "recall bias" present in case-control studies can be avoided.

Observational studies can provide evidence for an association between a putative exposure, or agent, and a particular disease. In a cohort study, the existence of an association is determined by comparing the occurrence of disease in those who are exposed to the factor of interest to its occurrence in those without the exposure—or those with a much lower level of exposure. The measure of association in a cohort study is called the *relative risk*. In a case-control study, one compares the occurrence of the exposure of interest between cases and controls. The measure of association summarizing this relationship is referred to as the *odds ratio*. If the relative risk or odds ratio is greater than 1.0 (no association), and the role of chance is deemed to be low, there is a positive association between the exposure and the disease. If the relative risk or odds ratio is below 1.0, this indicates that the exposure is inversely associated with the disease, possibly indicating a protective effect.

But what is an association? An association is merely a statistical relationship between two variables, similar to a correlation. If two variables are correlated, as one increases, the other increases. Every epidemiology and statistics textbook emphasizes that the existence of an association does not provide proof of causation. There are innumerable examples of correlations that have nothing to do with causation. In the 1950s statisticians pointed out that, internationally, sales of silk stockings tended to be highly correlated with cigarette consumption. Another example is that taller people tend to have higher IQs, but height is clearly not a cause of increased intelligence.

Finding a new association between an exposure and a disease, or physiologic state, is only the first step in a demanding process of obtaining the highest-quality data possible to confirm the existence of the association and to understand what it means. Does it represent a statistical fluke? Is an observed association between two factors merely due to their association with a third factor and thus merely a secondary phenomenon? How strong is the association? How consistently is it observed in different studies, and particularly in high-quality studies? Is it overshadowed by other, stronger and more convincing, associations? Is it consistent with a causal explanation? Is it in line with what is known regarding the biology of the disease?

Let's examine examples of associations that have been firmly established and accepted as causal. In the 1950s and 1960s both case-control and cohort studies showed that current smokers of cigarettes had between a ten- and twentyfold increased risk of developing lung cancer compared to those who had never smoked, while former smokers had a lesser but still palpable risk. In the 1970s a number of studies showed that women who used postmenopausal hormone therapy (which at that time tended to be high-dose estrogen) had roughly a fourfold increased risk of endometrial cancer. Other studies showed that heavy consumption of alcohol was associated with increased risk of cancers of the mouth and throat, with increased risks in the range of four- to sixfold.

These three associations have been confirmed by many subsequent studies and are among the solid findings we have concerning factors that have an effect on health. Examples like these represent success stories, where researchers addressing the same question pursued an initial association using different methods in different populations, and the resulting evidence has lined up to demonstrate that these are robust findings.

If one were to give a graphical presentation of the findings of many different studies on these questions, with a single point representing each study, one would see a cloud of dots—with some spread to be sure—in the quadrant indicating the existence of a substantial association.

It is crucial to realize, however, that not all associations are equal. Appreciating the distance traversed from an initial observation of an association to establishing that a specific factor or exposure is, in fact, likely to be a cause of disease is fundamental to understanding the confusion that pervades much of the reporting regarding results from observational studies. The success stories represent a miniscule fraction of the many questions—associations—that are studied, and must be studied, to uncover new and important evidence regarding the causes of disease. We must always keep in mind the denominator—in other words, the large number of questions that had to be explored in order to reach a solid new finding that makes a difference.

Science works by reducing the complexity of a biological system to what the researcher posits may be crucial players. In the simplest instance, one posits that exposure A is associated with disease B. In epidemiologic studies involving humans, this means examining the association between A and B in the population one has selected to study. The association between A and B can be represented by the arrow connecting them, as in figure 2.1. In the case of smoking and lung cancer, we have a strong exposure—that is to say, the average smoker may smoke roughly a pack of cigarettes per day for a period of more than forty years. Over decades, the repeated exposure of the lungs to the many toxins and carcinogens in tobacco smoke increases the likelihood of abnormal changes in the cells lining the airways and lungs, thereby increasing the chances that the smoker will develop lung cancer. Thus, in retrospect, based on hundreds of studies—epidemiologic, clinical, biochemical, and experimental—the association of cigarette smoking and lung cancer is now supported by a wealth of confirmatory evidence. So this is the basis for the statement that a current smoker has roughly a twentyfold increased risk of developing lung cancer.

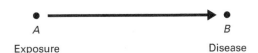

Figure 2.1
Association between an exposure and a disease.

What is too often lost sight of is that the established causal association between smoking and lung cancer is the result of decades of accumulated evidence. This strong association between a common exposure (roughly forty million Americans are still smokers) and a major cancer provides an important standard for gauging other reported associations. The two other exposures I mentioned above—use of postmenopausal hormones and heavy alcohol consumption—are also significant risk factors, although not as strong as smoking—and the associations observed with them are also credible.

Many of the research findings that get a great deal of media attention involve associations where the linkage between exposure A and disease, or physiologic state, B is preliminary and tenuous, and the observed association is much weaker than are those just mentioned. The one-line figure connecting an exposure and a disease, which are both isolated from their context, is hardly a realistic representation of what is involved. A more accurate representation would depict the many factors that are correlated with exposure A, the many other factors that may influence disease B, either positively or negatively, and the many intervening steps and linkages that are an integral part of the context in which exposure A may be associated with disease B. Figure 2.2 depicts this more complete picture.

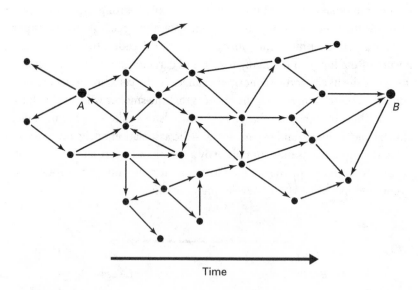

Figure 2.2
Any association we study is embedded in a thicket of other correlations.

In addition to the complexity of the linkages between a particular exposure and a disease, another problem is that other exposures are typically ignored to focus on the association of interest. To make this point more concrete, let's consider the situation of a researcher who is interested in the possible associations of human exposure to various chemicals in the environment on the risk of death and disease. This is an area of great interest to health researchers. However, the chemical pollutants that are studied are often correlated both with one another and with clinical variables, such as triglycerides, cholesterol, blood pressure, body mass index, and vitamin E levels, that are also associated with disease risk. This is shown in the "correlation globe" in figure 2.3. The lines connecting different points on the circle indicate correlations (either positive or negative) among the various environmental pollutants and clinical risk factors measured in blood or urine in the National Health and Nutrition Examination Survey between 1999 and 2006.[9]

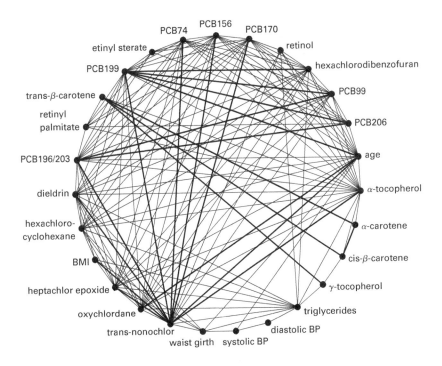

Figure 2.3
"Correlation globe" showing correlations among environmental pollutants and clinical variables in the National Health and Nutrition Examination Survey.
*Source*: By permission of John Ioannidis.

The figure drives home the importance of taking into account the many correlated exposures simultaneously to assess the importance of any specific factor, rather than isolating one factor, or a small number of factors, of interest and disregarding the complex nexus in which they are embedded. Many associations are there to be discovered; however, owing to the problem of correlation, and confounding, these associations tell us little about causation. Needless to say, the environmental and clinical factors shown in figure 2.3 represent only a small fraction of all potentially relevant factors.

In spite of what is written in textbooks, taught to graduate students, and explained in the best science journalism, researchers and laypeople alike are capable of slipping back into acting as if a *potential* association that is being studied represents a causal association—in other words, substituting the picture in figure 2.1 for that in figure 2.2. In many cases, the narrow focus on the question that interests the researcher and on the data he or she has collected crowds out attention to the many limitations of the study as well as to the context in which the findings should be interpreted. I will mention just a few common deficiencies, which raise questions about the validity of an observed association. First, often we are dealing with a one-time measurement of A, and the actual exposure is in many cases minute. Second, the single measurement may be temporally at a far remove from the occurrence of the putative effect (i.e., the disease or physiologic state). In other words, this is very different from the case of smoking, where, owing to its habitual nature, the exposure is both regular and substantial, and different from exposure to the Ebola virus, where the effects are apparent within a matter of days. Finally, in many studies the exposure of interest is considered in stark isolation from the many intervening and concomitant exposures that might modify or dwarf its effects. If one only considers the isolated association that one is interested in, one risks falling for the "illusion of validity" discussed in the previous chapter, and this blinkered focus can, in turn, blot out more important factors.

A recent example of the phenomenon of highlighting the association one is interested in and ignoring the all-important context and the nuances of the data is a paper by researchers at the University of California at Berkeley claiming an association of DDT exposure in utero and the development of breast cancer in women decades later.[10] The researchers used data from fifty-four years of follow-up of 20,754 pregnancies, resulting in 9,300 liveborn female offspring. Blood samples were obtained from the mothers during pregnancy and immediately after delivery. DDT levels in the mother's blood were compared between 118 breast cancer cases, diagnosed by age 52, and 354 controls. The authors reported that one of three isoforms of DDT was nearly fourfold higher in the blood of mothers of the breast cancer cases compared to that of mothers of controls. The point to keep in mind is that, even though the authors controlled for a number of factors in their analysis, the study only considered a one-time measurement of the factor of interest and related this measurement to the occurrence of disease some fifty years later. While it is conceivable that in utero exposure to DDT may influence a woman's risk of breast cancer, one has to step back and view the reported result in the context of all that has been passed over in the fifty-year interval separating the in utero measurement from the occurrence of disease. Although the authors adjusted for a number of characteristics of the *mothers*, their analysis ignored many intervening exposures and other factors that may influence both DDT levels and their endogenous effects, as well as factors that may influence breast cancer risk in the *daughters*. These include the daughter's postnatal exposure to DDT, age at menarche, age at first birth, how many children she has had, body weight, physical activity, breast-feeding history, alcohol consumption, and use of exogenous hormones. Thus while the study attracted widespread media attention, one has to realize how tenuous the result is. Like most studies of this kind, it raises more questions than it answers.

## A SURFEIT OF ASSOCIATIONS

According to the online bibliographic database PubMed, in 1969 the number of published scientific papers in the area of "epidemiology and cancer" was 625. This number increased steadily over the next forty-five years, reaching 12,030 in 2015, representing nearly a twentyfold increase. A search on the terms "environmental toxicology and cancer" yields many fewer papers—2 in 1969 and 423 in 2015—but a two-hundredfold increase. The enormous increase in publications in this area reflects the dramatic growth of the fields of epidemiology and environmental health sciences in academia, government and regulatory agencies, nongovernmental organizations, and industry.

A major asset in the conduct of epidemiologic research has been the establishment of large cohort studies. These represent enormous investments of government funding and of researchers' time required to design, implement, and monitor studies, many of which have tens or hundreds of thousands of participants. Such studies include information on a wide range of exposures and behaviors, including medical history, personal habits and behaviors, diet, and, increasingly, clinical and genetic information. Once a cohort is established, participants can be followed for decades, and new features can be added to the existing study. Modern technology, including bar-coding of samples and questionnaires, long-term storage of blood and other clinical samples, and computerized databases, has made possible the creation of immensely valuable repositories of data that can be used to address a potentially infinite number of questions concerning factors that influence health. There are now hundreds of cohort studies of different populations around the world designed to address different questions.

But there is another side to the existence of these large, rich databases. If one has information on, say, two hundred exposures and follows the population for years, ascertaining many different outcomes and considering different modifying factors, one has a very large number of associations to investigate. Such datasets make it possible to examine an almost infinite number of associations to see what turns up in the data. This is referred to as data dredging, or *deming*.[11] Want to see whether people who consume more broccoli have a lower incidence of ovarian cancer, or whether those with higher levels of BPA or some other contaminant in their blood or urine have a greater frequency of obesity, diabetes, or some other condition? One can have an answer in a couple of strokes of the keyboard. There is no end to the number of comparable questions one can address. Researchers who are funded to develop, maintain, and exploit these datasets have a strong incentive to publish the results of such analyses, even when the data to address the question are limited and the question itself has only a weak justification. Furthermore, graduate and postdoctoral students need to find new questions and to publish papers in order to establish themselves in the field. Owing to these incentives, some prominent cohort studies are the source of a huge number of publications each year. The ability afforded by these large cohort studies to address an almost infinite number of questions is captured in a cartoon that originally appeared in the *Cincinnati Enquirer* in 1997 (fig. 2.4).

An example of an area in which much work has been done but where results have been weak, inconsistent, and disappointing is the field of diet/nutrition and cancer. By the 1970s, based on geographical differences in cancer rates and animal experiments, researchers had surmised that many common cancers might be caused by excesses or deficiencies of diet. Since the 1980s thousands of epidemiologic studies have been published

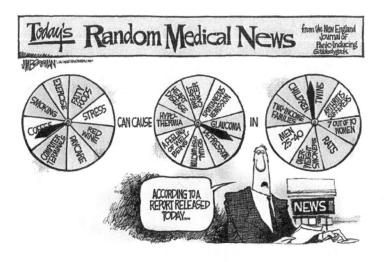

Figure 2.4
A very large number of associations can be generated from epidemiologic databases.
Cartoon by Jim Borgman. *Source*: Universal Uclick.

investigating this issue, and certain findings have garnered widespread
public attention. These include dietary fat and breast cancer; coffee intake
and various cancers; lycopene intake as a protective factor for prostate cancer; broccoli and other cruciferous vegetables as potential protective factors
for breast and other cancers; and many others. When one looks systematically at the results of these studies, however, very few associations stand up.
In its updated summary of the evidence on diet and cancer, the World Cancer Research Fund/American Institute for Cancer Research conducted a
detailed review of thousands of studies examining the association between
diet and cancer. The evidence regarding specific foods and beverages was
classified as "limited/suggestive," "probable," or "convincing." The only associations that were judged to be "convincing" were those of alcohol intake
with increased risk of certain cancers, of body weight with increased risk
of certain cancers, and of red meat intake with risk of colorectal cancer.[12]

Another approach to examining the accumulated evidence regarding diet and cancer was taken by Schoenfeld and Ioannidis, who noted
that associations with cancer risk or benefits have been claimed for most
food ingredients.[13] They randomly selected fifty foods or ingredients from

a popular cookbook and then searched the scientific literature for associations with cancer risk. What they found was that for most of the foods studied, positive associations were often counterbalanced by negative associations. Furthermore, the majority of reported associations were statistically significant. However, meta-analyses of these studies (that is, studies that combined the results of individual studies to obtain what amounts to a weighted average, which is more stable) produced much more conservative results: only 26 percent reported an increased or decreased risk. Furthermore, the magnitude of the associations shrank in meta-analyses from about a doubling, or a halving, of risk to no significant increase/decrease in risk. This suggests that "many single studies highlight implausibly large effects, even though evidence is weak." When examined in meta-analyses, the associations are greatly reduced.

## WHY MOST RESEARCH FINDINGS ARE FALSE

In recent years there has been growing awareness of biases and misconceptions affecting published studies in the area of biomedicine.[14] One figure, however, stands out for his prolific and penetrating research into the "research on research" in the area of health studies. John P. A. Ioannidis first attracted widespread attention with a 2005 article published in the *Public Library of Science Medicine* entitled "Why Most Published Research Findings are False." The paper caused a sensation and is the most frequently cited paper published in the journal. Actually, Ioannidis argues that the seemingly provocative assertion of the title should not come as a surprise. As he explains, the probability that a research finding is true depends on three factors: the "prior probability" of its being true; the statistical power of the study; and the level of statistical significance. The prior probability of its being true refers to the fact that, if there is some strong support for a hypothesis or for a causal association before one undertakes a study, this increases the probability of a new finding being true. "Statistical power" refers to the ability to detect an association, which is dependent on the sample size of the study and on the quality of the data. Finally, the level of statistical significance is the criterion for declaring a result "statistically significant"—that is, unlikely to be due to chance. Declaring a given result to be true when it is actually likely to be false is the result of *bias*. Bias has a different meaning from what we are used to in common parlance, where it suggests a moral failing or prejudice. With respect to research design, bias refers to any aspect of a study—its analysis, interpretation, or reporting—that systematically distorts the relationship one is examining. "Thus, with increasing bias, the chances that a research finding is true diminish considerably."[15]

The power of the approach taken by Ioannidis and colleagues comes from using statistics to survey the totality of findings on a given question to assess the quality of the data and the consistency and strength of the results. This approach provides the equivalent of a topographical map of the domain of studies on a given question. If a finding is real, it should be seen in studies of comparable quality and sample size that used similar methods of analysis. If the result is apparent only in weaker studies but not the stronger ones, then the association is probably wrong. If the results are inconsistent across studies of comparable quality, one must try to identify what factors account for this inconsistency. Rather than favoring those results suggesting a positive association, one can gain valuable insight by trying to explain such inconsistencies.

Only by examining the full range of studies on a given question and considering their attributes (sample size, quality of the measurements, rigor of the statistical analysis) and the strength and consistency of results across different studies, can one form a judgment of the quality of the evidence. Just as one has to look at large groups, or populations, to identify factors that may play a role in disease, so one has to examine the entire body of studies on a given question and the consistency and magnitude of the findings to make an assessment of their strength and validity.

In the *PLoS* paper, Ioannidis enumerated a number of different factors that increase the likelihood that a given result is false: (1) the smaller the size of the studies conducted in a given scientific field; (2) the smaller the "effect sizes" (that is, the smaller the magnitude of the association); (3) the greater the number and the lesser the selection of tested relationships in a scientific field; (4) the greater the flexibility in designs, definitions, outcomes, and analytical modes in a scientific field; (5) the greater the financial and other interests and prejudices in a scientific field; and (6) the "hotter" a scientific field (with more scientific teams involved). Notice that the factors influencing the likelihood of a false result range from the most basic design features (the size of the study) to sociological and psychological factors.

This approach to judging the credibility of the scientific evidence on a given question can be applied to vastly different content areas, and Ioannidis has collaborated with a large number of researchers in diverse fields to evaluate the evidence on many important questions. In hundreds of articles examining an extraordinary range of specialties and research questions—from etiology and treatment of specific diseases to the role of genetics, to the effectiveness of psychotherapy—Ioannidis and his collaborators have undertaken to map and analyze "an epidemic of false claims."[16]

A second paper by Ioannidis also published in 2005 asked the question: how often are high-impact clinical interventions that are reported in the literature later found to be wrong or found to be less impressive than indicated by the original report?[17] For this analysis, the author selected a total of forty-nine clinical research studies published in major clinical journals and cited more than one thousand times in the medical literature. He compared these papers to subsequently published studies of larger sample size and equal or superior quality. Sixteen percent of the original studies were contradicted by subsequent studies, and another 16 percent found effects that were stronger than those of the subsequent studies. Ioannidis concluded that it was not unusual for influential clinical results to be contradicted by later research or for researchers to report stronger effects than were subsequently confirmed.

Another major insight that has emerged from this work is that the quality and credibility of published results vary dramatically in different disciplines. Just as not all studies are equal in terms of quality, so not all disciplines are equal. For example, studies of the contribution of genetic variants to disease have become extremely rigorous owing to agreed-on standards for large populations and the requirement of replication. In contrast, epidemiologic studies of dietary and environmental factors tend to be much weaker and less credible. One analysis by Ioannidis and colleagues of ninety-eight meta-analyses of biomarker associations with cancer risk indicated that associations with infectious agents, such as *H. pylori*, hepatitis virus, and human papillomavirus, with risk of specific malignancies were "very strong and uncontestable," whereas associations of dietary factors, environmental factors, and sex hormones with cancer were much weaker.[18]

In hundreds of articles written with many different collaborators, Ioannidis has identified the pervasive occurrence of largely unquestioned biases operating in the medical literature. His work suggests how incorrect inferences can become entrenched in the literature and become accepted wisdom, and that it takes work to counteract this tendency. Some of the main themes that emerge in different contexts in this work are that initial findings with strong results tend to be followed by studies showing weaker results (dubbed the "Proteus phenomenon"); most true associations are inflated; even after prominent findings have been refuted, they continue to be cited as if they were true, and this can persist for years; limitations are not properly acknowledged in the scientific literature; most results in human nutrition research are implausible; and there is an urgent need for critical assessment and replication of biomedical findings. Ioannidis and colleagues conclude that new institutions and codes of research need to be devised in order to foster an improved research ecosystem.[19]

## ASSESSING CAUSALITY

Most questions that arise concerning human health cannot be answered by conducting a clinical trial. Therefore experimental proof is usually not a possibility, and most often we have to rely on observational studies. For the past forty years there has been an ongoing debate in the public health community regarding the extent to which causal inferences can be drawn from observational studies, and methods for improving the validity of inferences from epidemiologic studies have become much more sophisticated in the past two decades. In 1965 the British statistician Austin Bradford Hill published a landmark paper titled "The Environment and Disease: Association or Causation?" in which he discussed a number of considerations for use in judging whether an association was likely to be causal.[20] These are the strength of the association, consistency, specificity, temporality, biological gradient, plausibility, coherence, experimental evidence, and analogy. These have become enshrined as the Hill "criteria of judgment," although Hill never used the word "criteria" and never argued that a simple checklist could be used to make a definitive judgment about the causality of an association. Exceptions can be found to all of Hill's items.[21] Even fulfillment of all the "viewpoints" does not guarantee that an association is causal. In his influential paper, Hill actually emphasized the pitfalls of measurement error and overreliance on statistical significance in drawing conclusions about causality. However, in spite of his clear caveats and in spite of the improvement in epidemiologic methods for dealing with bias and error in epidemiologic studies, the "criteria of judgment" are still widely taught and widely invoked in the medical literature to assess the evidence on a given question.[22] Ironically, his "considerations" may be most appropriate when they are applied to questions where we have strong evidence from a number of different disciplines that support a causal association, as in the cases of cigarette smoking and lung cancer and human papillomavirus and cervical cancer.

Our ideas about causality derive from our early experience of the world.[23] And we tend to simplify by paying attention to the single most evident or the most proximate cause of some event. We do not tend to think in terms of multiple causes, but, as is true of historical events, disease conditions never have just one cause. In fact, even in the case of smoking and lung cancer, where we have a very strong, established cause, smoking by itself is not sufficient to cause the disease, since only one-seventh of smokers develop lung cancer. Similarly, in the case of infectious diseases, some people will not be susceptible by virtue of their immune competence, whereas others may be particularly susceptible because of poor nutritional status or poor resistance. Other chronic diseases like heart disease have a large number of component causes. What this means is that causality in the area of epidemiology is much more complex than our everyday notions allow for.

In the absence of a simple checklist that can be used to determine whether a given association is likely to be causal, the epidemiologists Ken Rothman and Sander Greenland have proposed an alternative to the invocation of Hill's "criteria."[24] They argue that careful exploration of the available data is necessary and that, in addition to considering the evidence that appears to support an association, one must explore the many pitfalls and biases in the study design and the data that could produce a spurious association. They opt for an intermediate position between those who unreservedly support the use of a checklist of causal criteria and those who reject it as having no value. According to Rothman and Greenland, "such an approach avoids the temptation to use causal criteria simply to bolster pet theories at hand, and instead allows epidemiologists to focus on evaluating competing causal theories using crucial observations."

The concluding paragraph of their article is worth quoting in full:

> Although there are no absolute criteria for assessing the validity of scientific evidence, it is still possible to assess the validity of a study. What is required is much more than the application of a list of criteria. Instead, one must apply thorough criticism, with the goal of obtaining a qualified evaluation of the total error that afflicts the study. This type of assessment is not one that can be done easily by someone who lacks the skills and training of a scientist familiar with the subject matter and the scientific methods that were employed. Neither can it be applied readily by judges in court, nor by scientists who either lack the requisite knowledge or who do not take the time to penetrate the work.[25]

Rothman and Greenland's prescription for unstintingly critical assessment of individual studies and, by implication, of the entire body of studies bearing on a specific question represents an ideal to which the field should aspire. There is no simple formula for assessing the evidence on a given topic. The evidence has to be evaluated on its own terms, taking into account all relevant findings and holding them up to scrutiny. It is painfully clear, however, that many scientific reports fall far short of critically evaluating the data they present. Being critical of one's own findings and of the work of others on a question in which one has a stake is a tall challenge and a commodity in short supply.

## STRONG INFERENCE

In spite of the many pitfalls and occasions for bias in observational studies, somehow science manages to make undreamed of advances. Rothman and Greenland point out that science has made impressive advances that were not arrived at through experimentation, and they cite the discovery of tectonic plates, the effects of smoking on human health, the evolution of species, and planets orbiting other stars as examples.[26] And there are many other examples relating to the health sciences. Two questions at the heart of this book are, first, how is it that extraordinary progress is made in solving certain problems, whereas in other areas little progress is made, and, second, why do instances of progress get so little attention, while those issues that gain attention often tend to be scientifically questionable?

Part of the answer lies in the nature of the scientific enterprise. Science is defined as "knowledge about, or study of, the natural world based on facts learned through experiments and observation." The Greek word for "to find" or "to discover" is *heuriskein*, and the word *heuristics* has made it into a common parlance to refer to techniques—such as "trial-and-error"— that lead to discovery. Use of the word heuristics implies that inherent in the scientific process is the fact that one cannot tell in advance where a given line of inquiry will lead, and that one doesn't know what one has found until one has found it. (This undoubtedly accounts for much of the excitement and exhilaration of science.)

At the same time, we have seen that often shortcuts—or simplified ideas—are resorted to in order to make sense of a difficult question, and these too have been referred to as "heuristics." The fact that the same word is used to refer both to the unpredictable process of arriving at solid new knowledge and to oversimplifications or false leads suggests how uncertain the process of scientific discovery is.

\* \* \*

Where do strong hypotheses come from, and how does one identify a productive line of inquiry? While there is no way to generalize, it is clear that being able to formulate a novel hypothesis requires a thoroughgoing, critical assessment of the existing evidence on a question. In this task, there are no shortcuts or general prescriptions that are applicable to all circumstances. There is only the coming to grips with the particulars of what is known about a question and formulating a picture of the terrain and evaluating the important features in order to identify gaps, reconcile conflicting findings, and come up with new connections.

Because we are dealing with complex, multifactorial diseases, such as breast cancer, heart disease, and Alzheimer's, it has to be understood that many alternative ideas must be explored, and most will not lead anywhere. This is not surprising, and there is no way to know in advance which approach will prove productive. However, the uncovering of new basic knowledge is likely to lead to a deeper understanding of a problem. Furthermore, progress is made in some areas and not in others. For example, striking progress has been achieved over the past thirty years in the treatment of breast cancer, whereas, in spite of an enormous amount that has been learned about the disease and its risk factors, we lack knowledge that would enable us to predict who will develop breast cancer or to prevent the disease.[27]

The critical assessment of evidence is part and parcel of coming up with new and better ideas. Often a field gets fixated on a particular idea, and this can stand in the way of fresh thinking and block the path to coming up with new ideas. There is a tendency for researchers to rework the same terrain over and over and produce studies that add little or nothing to what was done earlier. A prominent epidemiologist has referred to this as "circular epidemiology."[28] Another epidemiologist, who has been involved in the study of a number of high-profile environmental exposures, has stressed the importance of knowing when research on a topic has reached the point of diminishing returns, so that resources and energy can be devoted to other, more fruitful avenues.[29]

What can one say about the attitudes and methods that lead to new ways of seeing a problem and making real progress? Of course, it is not possible to be programmatic or prescriptive. However, when one examines specific problems and what their study has yielded—as in the four case studies that make up the core of this book—there are characteristics and attitudes that appear to have played a major role in making possible dramatic progress. On the other hand, other areas of study have characteristics that help explain why a question can continue to be a source of concern and to attract research with little prospect of making progress.

The first, and least teachable, faculty or characteristic that can lead to transformative insight into a problem is being observant and being able to see things that are in front of one's eyes, or in the data on a question. We will see striking examples of this in later chapters. Second, a productive hypothesis often stems from a *strong signal*. For example, why are the rates of a particular disease dramatically higher in one geographic region or in one social or ethnic group than another? Why has a disease increased, or decreased, in frequency? Or, if one is interested in a specific exposure, it makes sense to study a population or occupational group that has a high exposure to see if one can document effects in that population. These kinds of questions have often provided the starting point for epidemiologic investigations. Third, one must characterize the phenomenon under study in all its particularity, defining a disease entity and documenting its natural history, relevant exposures and cofactors, and environmental conditions associated with it. Fourth, it is important to look for contradictions in the evidence, for things that don't fit. This can lead one to modify a hypothesis and sharpen it, or to reject it in part or in its totality. Fifth, a particularly fruitful tactic is to make connections between phenomena that have not previously been brought into relation. We will see examples of this in the last two case studies. Finally, one has to be willing to question the most basic prevailing assumptions and take a fresh look at the evidence, as Abraham Wald did when examining the pattern of damage on the returning Lancasters. This can lead to overturning of the reigning dogma, as occurred when Barry Marshall and Robin Warren demonstrated that, contrary to entrenched opinion, bacteria could grow in the stomach, in spite of the high acidity. And they proceeded to demonstrate that bacterial infection with *Helicobacter pylori* is a major cause of stomach ulcers and stomach cancer. Their work completely overturned the prevailing wisdom that ascribed stomach ulcers to psychological stress and to eating spicy food. Something similar occurred when Harald zur Hausen rejected the idea that herpes simplex virus was a cause of cervical cancer and turned his attention to a totally difference class of viruses, the papillomaviruses.

## THE METHOD OF EXCLUSION

Although intangible factors like instinct and luck can play a role in identifying a productive line of inquiry, too little attention is given to the practice of rigorous reasoning in considering competing hypotheses and excluding possibilities. In 1964 the biophysicist John R. Platt of the University of Chicago published a paper in the journal *Science* entitled "Strong Inference"—a paper that should be read by anyone with an interest in what distinguishes successful science.[30] Platt argued that certain systematic methods of scientific thinking can produce much more rapid progress than others. He saw the enormous advances in molecular biology and high-energy physics as examples of what this approach can yield. He wrote, "On any new problem, of course, inductive inference is not as simple and certain as deduction, because it involves reaching out into the unknown." "Strong inference" involves (1) devising alternative hypotheses; (2) devising a crucial experiment that will exclude one or more hypotheses; (3) carrying out the experiment so as to get a clean result; and (4) repeating the procedure, devising further hypotheses to refine the possibilities that remain. Of course, in epidemiology and public health we are not talking about carrying out experiments. Nevertheless, Platt's prescription for a rigorous approach to the evidence is highly relevant to epidemiology and very much in line with Rothman and Greenland's and Ioannidis's prescription for unstinting, critical evaluation of the biases and errors that afflict studies on a given question.

Platt aligns himself with Francis Bacon, who emphasized the power of "proper rejections and exclusions," and Karl Popper, who posited that a useful hypothesis is one that can be falsified. And he goes on to cite the "second great intellectual invention," "the method of multiple hypotheses" put forward by the geologist T. C. Chamberlin of the University of Chicago in 1890. Chamberlin advocated the formulation of multiple hypotheses as a means of guarding against one's natural inclination to become emotionally invested in a single hypothesis.[31] This approach of pursuing evidence that bears on multiple hypotheses makes it possible to adjudicate between competing hypotheses. Following Chamberlin, Platt argues that adopting the method of entertaining multiple hypotheses leads to a collective focus on the work of disproof and exclusion and transcends conflicts between scientists holding different hypotheses.[32]

Platt is unsparing in his assessment of those who collect and enumerate data without formulating clear hypotheses:

Today we preach that science is not science unless it is quantitative. We substitute correlations for causal studies, and physical equations for organic reasoning. Measurements and equations are supposed to sharpen thinking, but, in my observation, they more often tend to make the thinking noncausal and fuzzy. They tend to become the object of scientific manipulation instead of auxiliary tests of crucial inferences.

What I am saying is that, in numerous areas that we call science, we have come to like our habitual ways, and our studies that can be continued indefinitely. We measure, we define, we compute, we analyze, but we do not exclude. And this is not the way to use our minds most effectively or to make the fastest progress in solving scientific questions.

The man to watch, the man to put your money on is not the man who wants to make "a survey" or a "more detailed study" but the man with the notebook, the man with the alternative hypotheses and the crucial experiments, the man who knows how to answer your question of disproof and is already working on it.[33]

Platt distinguished two types of science: science that uses a systematic method to identify the next step and make progress and science that is stuck in place and has no strategy to make exclusions and to move forward. But his focus is on the scientific establishment alone, and, tellingly, he has nothing to say about the interaction between science and the wider society. Nevertheless, one has no trouble imagining what he would think of scientists who resort to the court of public opinion to gain support for the importance of their work, rather than coming to grips with the totality of the evidence and subjecting a favored hypothesis to unstinting criticism. It is to the question of the interaction between science touching on high-profile health issues and the wider society that we must turn in the following chapter.

# 3

# When Risk Goes Viral
## *Biases and Bandwagons*

---

The resulting mass delusions may last indefinitely, and they may produce wasteful or even detrimental laws and policies.

—TIMUR KURAN AND CASS SUNSTEIN

---

## SCIENCE AND SOCIETY

To begin to make sense of the conflicting scientific findings and disputes bedeviling issues associated with public health, we need to start by recognizing that discourse about health risks and health benefits generated by biomedicine is deeply embedded in society. In a democracy, scientific research ultimately depends on support of citizen taxpayers and public opinion, which influence political support in the Congress and the budgetary process. There are interactions between the scientific community and the public sphere, and the relationship between science and society is reciprocal and complex, operating on many levels. Different groups—scientists (who themselves fall into different disciplines with different points of view), regulators, health officials, lay advocates, journalists, businessmen, lawyers—are shaped by different backgrounds and motivated by different beliefs and agendas. Depending on the issue at hand, the interests of these parties may conflict or may align and reinforce one another.

There is a busy "traffic" in scientific findings regarding health between the various sectors of society. Figure 3.1 gives a schematic representation of how the findings of scientific studies are embedded in society and can be viewed as being at the center of a set of concentric circles. The encircling

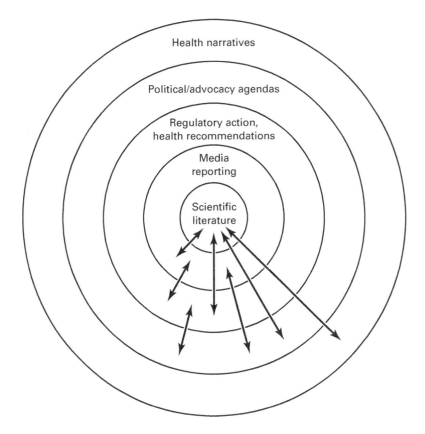

Figure 3.1
Schematic representation of interactions between scientific findings and the different communities that use them.

rings represent different "audiences" or communities, each with its own "reading"—or, more often, multiple readings—of the scientific evidence. As one moves outward from the center, the technical information at the center needs to be "translated" and adjusted to a particular audience. Translation for the news media takes one form; translation for the regulatory community takes another. Thus there are effects that radiate outward from one ring to another, as well as effects that skip an intervening ring. The information from individual circles can also combine and have a joint effect. For example, the combination of scientific findings plus media reporting and resulting public concern can set regulatory action in motion. Additionally, the three innermost circles acting in concert can shape the narrative—or competing narratives—that takes hold in the society at large on a particular question. But there are also feedbacks from the outer rings toward the center. Scientists are keenly aware that their work has effects beyond the scientific community, and this awareness can influence what research they undertake and how they interpret their findings. These bidirectional interactions are indicated by the two-headed arrows.

## REPORTING OF RISKS IN THE MEDIA

Media reporting of the results of scientific studies bearing on health risks exerts an influence in a class of its own. In recent years there has been an explosion in the number of media channels beyond newspapers, magazines, and television networks. The proliferation of websites, blogs, forums, "feeds," and television channels provides a constant stream of "content" tailored to the interests and orientations of consumers. This in turn has led to an increasing fragmentation or "cantonization" of the news.

The staples of media reporting are stories that have the appearance of being relevant to our lives. Thus a scientific finding that suggests an association between an exposure alleged to affect the general population and a disease is more likely to gain news coverage than findings from a negative study. Many players in the media see it as their mission, as well as a business necessity, to awaken interest in "new developments." They can't afford to devote resources to putting a research finding in context or reporting on the long slog of research on obscure topics, because this does not attract most readers or viewers. Thus much media reporting is the antithesis of a critical assessment of what the reported finding may actually mean. The implicit justification for these news items is that they provide information that will be of interest and of use to the public. But many, if not most, of these reports are simply misleading or wrong and convey "information" that is of no conceivable use.

It is not that there is no high-quality reporting in the area of health and health risks. On the contrary, there are many outstanding sources of informed and critical reporting on these issues. However, there are two problems. First, this more solid and more thoughtful journalism exists on a different plane from the much more salient reports that make headlines, and it cannot compete with the latter. Second, those who avail themselves of these more informed sources of information do so because they are looking for reliable information on complex and difficult questions. Thus this type of journalism is, to a large extent, preaching to the converted.

When a health-related issue is catapulted into the spotlight, it takes on a special status. The French sociologist of science Bruno Latour has taken an extreme and controversial view of "scientific facts" that is useful by virtue of its emphasis on the interpenetration of science and society.[1] Latour refers to objects of scientific study as *hybrids* and argues that there is no such thing as a pure scientific fact that can be dissociated from its social context and the technology used to study it. For example, according to Latour, a natural phenomenon, such as a virus, cannot be dissociated from the observations, concepts, and apparatus used to measure and characterize it. Beyond this, he argues that the way in which "facts" are disseminated into the public sphere is inseparable from the many associations that accrete around them. Whatever one ultimately thinks of Latour's view of science, his concept of "hybrids" is useful and apt in reference to the way in which scientific findings concerning public health risks get shaped in the public arena.

For whatever reasons, we tend to underestimate the power that such ideas have when they take hold in the wider society. To give just one example of what I mean, consider the widespread concern about the dangers of low-frequency electromagnetic fields (EMFs) that arose in the late 1970s and reached its apogee in the mid-1990s but still persists today. These fields are produced by electric current carried by power lines and generated by electrical appliances and motors, and as such are virtually ubiquitous in modern societies. However, the energy from these fields is extremely weak and falls off rapidly with increasing distance from the source. Given the a priori implausibility of these weak fields having dramatic effects on human health,[2] the way in which the issue was often dramatized for television audiences is not without significance. Typically, when a scientist appeared on the nightly news to discuss findings from the latest study, he would invariably be filmed against the backdrop of ominous-looking 735-kilovolt transmission lines. Whatever the validity of the reported findings—and these studies have been recognized as having serious flaws—the clear and effective message conveyed to the viewer was that there was a threat. The intense concern and uncertainty surrounding the question of the effects of these fields on health led to the conducting of hundreds of scientific studies and lawsuits to force electric utilities to relocate power lines. Although the scientific and regulatory communities have largely dismissed a risk from EMFs encountered in everyday life, many people, including some scientists, continue to this day to believe that there is a health risk.[3]

## KEY FACTORS AFFECTING THE INTERPRETATION OF
## SCIENTIFIC STUDIES

Textbooks of epidemiology routinely discuss a range of basic concepts relating to the conduct and interpretation of epidemiologic studies, such as measurement of disease occurrence, risk factors, measures of association, study design, the role of chance, statistical significance, confounding, bias, and sample size, and how these factors can affect the validity of the results. Understanding these concepts as well as the statistical methods used in analyzing epidemiologic studies is part of the competence that epidemiologists acquire in the course of their training. However, other factors that can influence the conduct and interpretation of epidemiologic studies—and biomedical studies generally—tend to get less attention because they have less to do with technical matters and more to do with "softer" issues, including how the data are interpreted, what limitations are acknowledged, how the findings are placed in the context of a larger narrative, what other studies are cited, what contrary evidence is discussed, and even less tangible factors, like philosophical and political orientation. Some considerations are so general and applicable to any scientific endeavor that they escape mention, even though there is ample evidence that they represent cognitive pitfalls and need to be taken seriously (e.g., the danger of becoming wedded to one's hypothesis; favoring certain findings and disregarding others that don't fit with one's position; having an investment in a particular result; allowing a political or ideological position to color one's interpretation of the data; ignoring countervailing evidence).

In this section I describe some of the features of the landscape in which research concerning health risks is interpreted in order to give a more realistic picture of the tools scientists have at their disposal, the limitations of the kinds of studies that are done, and the principles, concepts, and distinctions that come into play when interpreting research results and communicating them to the wider public. This will help us to understand how bias and subjective motivations can creep into the presentation of research findings and their dissemination to the society at large. The remainder of the chapter will explore how a distorted account of the scientific evidence can be amplified by cognitive biases operating in the wider society, resulting in costly scares and ill-conceived policies and regulations.

We have seen that the associations reported in epidemiologic and environmental studies are not always what they appear to be at first glance, and that the identification of a new association is only the beginning of a long process requiring better measurements and improved study designs to verify the linkages that underlie the association. Most initial associations do not stand up to this process. If the interpretation of associations is challenging and treacherous for scientists, once news of an association emerges into the public arena, the association can be transformed into something very different from what the scientific evidence supports and can take on a life of its own.

## ASSOCIATION VERSUS CAUSATION

As we saw in the previous chapter, we depend on observational studies to identify risk factors or protective factors associated with disease in humans. The associations reported in epidemiologic studies are simply correlations, and it is an axiom in epidemiology, as well as in philosophy going back to David Hume, that "association does not prove causation." Many phenomena are correlated and tend occur together without one causing the other. In addition, an observed association could be due to chance, confounding, or bias in the design of the study. These are things that students of epidemiology learn at the outset and that textbooks emphasize. However, something strange can happen when researchers publish a scientific paper examining the association of exposure X with health condition Y. In spite of the acknowledged limitations of the data and the awareness that one is examining associations, the message can be conveyed, either more or less overtly, that the data suggest a causal association. It appears to be difficult for researchers to study something that has to do with health and disease without going beyond what the data warrant.[4] If researchers can slip into this way of interpreting and presenting the results of their studies, it becomes easier to understand how journalists, regulators, activists of various stripes, self-appointed health gurus, promoters of health-related foods and products, and the public can make the unwarranted leap that the study being reported provides evidence of a causal relationship and therefore is worthy of our interest.

## DOSE, TIMING, AND THE PROPERTIES OF THE AGENT

Another axiom, which is the cornerstone of toxicology, is that "the dose makes the poison." The magnitude of one's exposure matters. This is true of micronutrients, such as iron, copper, selenium, and zinc, which our bodies need in minute quantities to make red blood cells and to manufacture enzymes, but which, taken in large amounts, are highly toxic. It is also true of lifestyle and personal exposures, such as cigarette smoking and consuming alcoholic beverages, and medications, as well as pollutants in the environment. Many toxins and carcinogens exhibit a dose-response relationship: that is, as the exposure increases, so too does the observed toxic or carcinogenic effect. Even compounds and foods we think of as healthy can be lethal when consumed in excess. For example, we need beta-carotene obtained from carrots and other vegetables and fruits for our bodies to make vitamin A. However, consuming carrots in excess can lead to the skin turning orange from hypercarotenosis and eventually to death. Similarly, consumption of excessive amounts of water can lead to an electrolyte imbalance and heart failure. Some compounds are much more toxic than others, and even minute amounts can have lethal effects—for example, polonium-210, ricin, and methyl mercury. In addition to the dose, different compounds have vastly different potencies, as I will discuss in relation to "endocrine disrupting chemicals." All this, of course, needs to be taken into account when evaluating an exposure. Nevertheless, what is noteworthy and disturbing is how frequently scientists examining an exposure of concern to the public (which, in many cases, was initiated in the first place by a scientific study) can ignore the issues of dose and potency or imply that they are seeing an effect of an exposure at a dose that is so low as to make the claimed effect questionable. Although modern technology gives us the ability to measure the amount of a compound in a sample down to parts per billion, this does not necessarily mean that trace exposures are having detectable health effects.

It should also be mentioned that the same compound can have very different effects depending on the timing of exposure. For example, it is now clear that estrogen given to women close to the onset of menopause increases the risk of breast cancer, whereas when given to women who are five or more years beyond menopause, estrogen decreases the risk of breast cancer.[5]

Finally, the nature of the agent being studied also needs to be taken into account. Radiofrequency energy and microwaves are many orders of magnitude weaker in energy than X-rays or ultraviolet radiation, both of which can damage DNA. This doesn't mean that radiofrequency and microwave energy do not merit study in terms of their potential health effects. But it does mean that, in studying them, one needs to be aware of the fact that one is likely to be dealing with more subtle and difficult-to-detect effects. Similar considerations apply to the study of "endocrine disrupting chemicals" in the environment. For example, the chemical BPA can act as a weak estrogen, but its potency is many orders of magnitude less than that of the natural estrogen estradiol. Again, it is striking how often, in scientific studies of health effects of such agents, these considerations are lost sight of.

## FALSE POSITIVE RESULTS

It is fair to say that researchers are motivated to identify relationships that play an *important* role in health and disease. Few researchers are likely to devote years to demonstrating that some factor does *not* play an important role in disease. Furthermore, if a study is suggestive of a weak association, or if a subgroup within the study population shows an association, there is an understandable tendency to not want to discount what could be an indication of a real risk. A small risk applied to a large population can translate into a substantial number of cases of disease. However, at the same time, an emphasis on blips in the data can mean giving undue weight to what only appears to be a positive result. Marcia Angell, a former editor of the *New England Journal of Medicine*, has said that "authors and investigators are worried that there's a bias against negative studies. And so they'll try very hard to convert what is essentially a negative study into a positive study by hanging on to very, very small risks or seizing on one positive aspect of a study which is by and large negative."[6]

One of the consistent findings of the studies conducted by Ioannidis and colleagues is that there are many more statistically significant positive findings reported in the medical literature than would be expected based on the ability to detect true findings. Nevertheless, the issue of false positives has been a topic of heated debate among researchers.[7]

What is beyond dispute is that positive results spur other researchers to attempt to confirm an association, and this process can lead to cascades of research findings that may be weakly suggestive of an association but largely spurious. What is also beyond dispute is that such false positive findings are likely to get attention from the media and, in some cases, the regulatory community. And this can lead to "availability cascades" in the wider society.[8]

## POSITIVE FINDINGS GET MORE ATTENTION THAN FINDINGS OF NO RELATIONSHIP

Positive findings linking an exposure to a disease are a valuable commodity and are of interest to other researchers, health and regulatory agencies, the media, and the general public. Where such findings are confirmed and become established as important influences on health (e.g., smoking and lung cancer; human papillomavirus and cervical cancer; obesity and diabetes), they have enormous importance for public health and may provide the means for reducing the toll of disease and death. However, research routinely generates positive findings that have a very different status. Many are weak or inconsistent findings that may conflict with other lines of evidence. Yet, in the researcher's eye, the preliminary positive finding may point to a new and important risk.

It is simply a fact of human nature that positive findings get more attention than findings of no relationship obtained in studies of comparable quality. And this applies to researchers, regulators, the media, and the general public. Positive associations appear to be more psychologically satisfying than studies that show no effect. They give us something to hold on to; they give us the illusion of knowledge on issues where we are eager for clear-cut information. Perhaps for these reasons, positive findings seem more credible—they feel truer than findings of no effect. Thus there is an important asymmetry between reports showing an effect and those showing no effect. This asymmetry is synonymous with bias.

### "HAZARD" VERSUS "RISK"

A crucial distinction lurking in the background in the assessment of health risks but rarely made explicit is that between hazard and risk. A *hazard* is a potential source of harm or adverse health effects. In contrast, *risk* is the likelihood that exposure to a hazard causes harm or some adverse effect.[9] The drain cleaner underneath one's sink is a hazard, but it will pose a risk only if one drinks it or gets it on one's hands. Thus a hazard's potential to pose a risk of detectable effects is realized only under specific circumstances, namely, sufficiently frequent exposure to a sufficient dose for a sufficient period of time. The confusion between hazard and risk afflicts many scientific publications and, particularly, regulatory "risk assessments." The most glaring example of this is the International Agency for Research on Cancer (IARC), an arm of the World Health Organization that publishes influential assessments of carcinogens in its series "IARC Monographs on the Evaluation of Carcinogenic Risks to Humans." In spite of the reference to "risk" in the title, IARC actually is concerned only with hazard and not with risk.[10] In other words, any evidence—whether from animal experiments, studies in humans, or mechanistic studies in the laboratory—that a compound or agent might be carcinogenic is emphasized in IARC's assessment, no matter what the magnitude of risk involved or the relevance to actual human exposure. This explains how in October 2015 the agency was able to classify processed meats, such as bacon, sausage, and salami, as "known human carcinogens," in the same category as tobacco, asbestos, and arsenic.[11]

## PUBLICATION BIAS

Publication bias refers to the fact that studies finding no evidence of an association between an exposure and a disease are less likely to be submitted for publication and, if submitted, are less likely to be published. Scientific and medical journals have a bias in favor of publishing positive and "interesting" findings. This is a well-documented phenomenon. Publication bias is simply the result of positive findings being more likely to be published. If carefully executed studies that produce "null" results (i.e., no support for the examined association) are not published, this distorts the scientific record and produces a skewed picture. Recently, the importance of publishing well-executed studies that report "null" findings has been gaining attention at the highest levels of the science establishment.[12]

## THE "MAGNIFYING GLASS EFFECT" OR BLINKERING EFFECT

Research and regulation tend to address risks one at a time, rather than placing a putative risk in the context of other risks that may be more important or considering countervailing effects of other exposures that may offset them. In this way, the risk that is focused on becomes the whole world and can blot out consideration of other, potentially more important risk factors that should be taken into account. A good example of this is the case with regard to "endocrine disrupting chemicals," where much of the research has had a narrow focus and has ignored factors, such as the recent increase in obesity, that could be expected to dwarf any effect of the exposure under study.[13] By focusing on risks one at time, isolated from their relevant context, one forgoes the opportunity to put them in perspective and make sense of them. This bias has been popularized in the adage, "When your only tool is a hammer, everything looks like a nail." A *New Yorker* cartoon

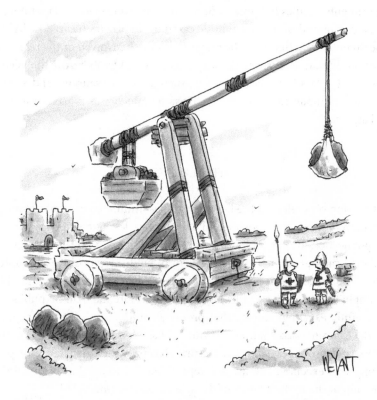

*"When your only tool is a trebuchet, every problem looks like a siege."*

Figure 3.2
Cartoon by Christopher Weyant.
*Source*: The New Yorker Collection/The Cartoon Bank.

(fig. 3.2) has cleverly refreshed this insight by transposing it to the Middle Ages. Another name for this blinkering effect is confirmation bias.

## THE PUBLIC IS SENSITIZED TO CERTAIN KINDS OF THREATS

We are predisposed to want to identify external causes rather than focusing on things closer to home—personal behaviors that we might be able to do more about. Studies by the psychologist Paul Slovic and others have shown that certain types of risks have much more salience for the public than others.[14] In general, threats that are invisible and not under our control (such as ionizing radiation or trace amounts of chemicals in food and water) tend to elicit a strong reaction from the public. Strikingly, other exposures that are much more important at the population level, such as cigarette smoking, weight gain, excessive alcohol consumption, and excessive sun exposure, do not elicit anywhere near the same reaction. This may be because we have the illusion that they are under our control but also because they are widespread and familiar—they have been "domesticated," so to speak. Thus news reports based on scientific studies implying that we and our children are being poisoned by chemicals in our water and food or being threatened by "radiation" from power lines and cell phone masts strike an exposed nerve.

## THE EXISTENCE OF AN ALARMED AND SENSITIZED PUBLIC IS USEFUL TO SCIENTISTS AND REGULATORS

When a question arises about the potential contribution of some environmental exposure to human health, the ability to obtain funds to conduct research depends in theory on the strength of the scientific case one can make for the value of the proposed study. Obtaining funding from the National Institutes of Health—by far the largest source of grant support for scientific research on health—is extremely competitive, and only a small percentage of submitted proposals are successful. However, if the media has picked up a question and made it a focus of public concern, this can influence the perception of the value of the proposed research. Special programs can be set up within federal agencies to focus attention on the topic, and in some cases special funds are even earmarked for research on it. The creation of a program within an agency, or supported by several agencies, gives the topic a special status. Furthermore, elevating a potential risk in this way sends a message to the public, since if something is being studied in this way, "it must be important." This is what happened with DDT/PCBs and breast cancer and with electromagnetic fields and breast cancer in the 1990s, and something similar happened with "endocrine disruption" in the 2000s. Testifying at a meeting of the California Air Resources Board regarding proposed regulation of diesel emissions, the University of California at Irvine air pollution researcher Robert Phalen commented, "It benefits us personally to have the public be afraid, even if these risks are trivial."[15]

At the same time, it is important to recognize that, in some circumstances, agencies have set up programs to support high-quality research to address a high-profile issue. This is what happened at the Food and Drug Administration and the Environmental Protection Agency in funding studies to elucidate population exposure to BPA as well as the pharmacokinetics of the chemical in animals and humans.

## ADVOCACY AND POLITICAL CORRECTNESS

As the role of science has grown in the sphere of public policy, advocacy for a specific policy position has become increasingly prevalent among scientists. Whether the issue is exposure to trace amounts of contaminants in the environment, smokers' access to potentially less harmful products that can replace cigarettes, concern about the role of certain foods and beverages in obesity, or something else, an adherence to a particular policy position can color one's reading of the science. This poses a serious threat to science, which must be independent of the personal beliefs and predilections of scientists.

On certain topics scientists, advocates, and members of the public can invoke the moral high ground by claiming that particular findings are beneficial for human health and society and that anyone who questions the solidity of the scientific evidence for a claim can be characterized as not having the public's best interests at heart. This is a form of political correctness and has been referred to as "white hat bias."[16] Mark Cope and David Allison described the use of this strategy to assert that intake of nutritively sweetened beverages disposed toward obesity and that breastfeeding provided protection against obesity, claims that, according to them, are not supported by the evidence. The authors documented instances in which results that are "politically correct" were more likely to be accepted by scientists and that findings "that do not agree with prevailing opinion may not be published." According to the authors, the bias was also reflected in inaccurate descriptions of results of studies to make them conform to the desired view.

## THE PEER-REVIEW SYSTEM

The peer-review system is supposed to serve as a bulwark against the publication of flawed and misleading research. However, all that stands between the publication of a poor piece of work and the public are journal editors and the peer reviewers, who agree to donate their time to evaluate a paper for publication. As is true of any system dependent on human beings, peer review is imperfect. It is only as good as the critical acumen that editors and reviewers bring to the task, and there are inevitable failures, namely, papers that get published that should never have been published.

The quality of review is variable. Often reviewers are insufficiently critical, and this can lead to the acceptance of papers that should have been rejected outright or accepted only after further evidence was provided in support of the conclusions or a fuller discussion of the limitations was provided. The work of John Ioannidis and others has underscored the poor quality of much of what gets published, even in highly respected medical journals.

And the sad truth is that virtually anything—no matter how bad—can get published somewhere. When a paper deals with a topic that has received widespread publicity and caused public alarm, this may have the effect of lowering the threshold for publication. In other words, to the extent that the reviewers and editors were aware that the paper was weak and its results questionable, they may have overridden these reservations on the grounds that the paper was on a topic of great interest and would stimulate further research. Finally, the standards for what is publishable and the level of scientific rigor and overall quality may be lower in certain areas, such as environmental health, where there is great public and media interest, as opposed to other research areas that do not evoke the same level of interest.[17]

In 1998 the British journal *Lancet* published a paper by the surgeon Andrew Wakefield purporting to show that children who had received the measles, mumps, and rubella (MMR) vaccine developed intestinal problems and autism. The paper's publication represents a staggering failure of peer review. It was reviewed by six peer reviewers and the editor, none of whom saw any reason not to publish it. In retrospect, it is hard to understand how anyone could think that any conclusion could be drawn from a series of twelve cases. Nevertheless, it took twelve years for the journal to retract the paper, and it was only due to the persistence of an investigative reporter that the fraud perpetrated by Wakefield was uncovered.[18] The disastrous effects of this paper are still very much with us. While the Wakefield case represents an extreme example, much that is published has not been held to a very high standard.

## CONFLICTS OF INTEREST

Today, when one submits a paper to a biomedical journal, one is routinely asked to declare any potential "conflicts of interest." This practice began in the 1990s owing to an increasing awareness that the reporting of results might be distorted due to influence of the sponsor of the research. At the outset this concern applied first and foremost to studies funded by industry, including the pharmaceutical, chemical, and tobacco industries. There is no question that there is the potential for abuse when the research findings may conflict with the interests of the commercial sponsor. In 1993, however, the epidemiologist Ken Rothman pointed out that financial conflicts of interest are only the most obvious, and therefore the easiest to spot instances of factors that could distort the research process.[19] Rothman argued that political, ideological, and professional motives could also affect the reporting of results. Since it is impossible to assess all the psychological and ideological factors that could influence the presentation of one's results, he proposed that a piece of work should be evaluated on its merits rather than on extrinsic factors. More recently, others have argued that nonfinancial conflicts of interest may be more important than financial ones.[20] Still, alleged financial conflicts of interest as well as ad hominem arguments are routinely used to counter opponents in controversies involving human health.

Ironically, the emphasis on financial relationships has created a situation in which advocates with strong partisan views who are aligned with a cause routinely declare "no conflict of interest" because it does not fit the prevailing narrow definition. This state of affairs underscores how deeply subjective factors and attitudes are intertwined with the reporting of results of scientific studies.

## THE DANGER OF BELIEVING ONE'S HYPOTHESIS

Science is propelled by new ideas, or hypotheses, that represent attempts to answer important questions by building on what is known, collecting new data, and making new connections. Once a worthwhile hypothesis is formulated, all that matters is to collect the most informative data possible to either support or refute it. Progress can be made only by bringing the best data to bear on the hypothesis. The new data may provide unqualified support for the hypothesis, require modification of the hypothesis, or flat

out contradict the hypothesis. Progress depends on the researcher's maintaining a tension between attachment to his or her idea and willingness to
be ruthlessly critical in evaluating the data that bear on it. One has to consider the evidence that goes counter to the hypothesis as well as that which
supports it.[21] A strong hypothesis is one that stands up to strong tests to
disprove it. The UCLA epidemiologist Sander Greenland has given a penetrating formulation of this tension: "There is nothing sinful about going
out and getting evidence, like asking people how much do you drink and
checking breast cancer records. There's nothing sinful about seeing if the
evidence correlates. There's nothing sinful about checking for confounding
variables. The sin comes in in believing a causal hypothesis is true because
your study came up with a positive result, or believing the opposite because
your study was negative."[22]

We are all susceptible to being fooled by ideas that appear to offer an
explanation for a mysterious phenomenon we are eager to understand. That
is why we require science—the careful, painstaking work of excluding alternative explanations and verifying each link in the causal chain as a safe-
guard against error. If scientists are susceptible to eliding these distinctions
and believing in their hypotheses, it is hardly surprising that the media and
the public are susceptible to the same slippage.

## THE PRECAUTIONARY PRINCIPLE

In the past few decades it has become routine for the so-called precautionary principle to be invoked whenever a question arises regarding the impact of a potential threat to health or the environment. The precautionary
principle or precautionary approach to risk management states that if an
action or policy has a suspected risk of causing harm to the public or the
environment, in the absence of scientific consensus that the action or policy is not harmful, the burden of proof that it is *not* harmful falls on those
taking the action.[23] The principle implies that there is a social responsibility
to protect the public from exposure to harm, when scientific investigation
has found a plausible risk. Since the 1980s the precautionary principle has
been adopted by the United Nations (World Charter for Nature, 1982) and
the European Commission of the European Union (2000) and has been
incorporated into many national legal systems.

In spite of its prominence in discussions of novel exposures and their effects on health and the environment, as the extensive literature on the topic

makes clear, there are numerous problems with this principle, which sounds so reasonable and commonsensical. First, the precautionary principle is difficult to define, and there are numerous interpretations that are incompatible with one another.[24] Second, it does not provide a clear guide to action, and it encourages taking a narrow view of risks, rather than considering them in context, together with alternatives, mitigation, trade-offs, and costs versus benefits.[25] Third, where there is disagreement among scientists and regulatory bodies regarding the existence of a risk to the public, those who believe the evidence pointing to a risk are apt to invoke the precautionary principle as a means of mobilizing public opinion. Finally, application of the principle tends to provoke public anxiety and can end up causing harm.

It is hard to quarrel with the maxim that "it's better to be safe than sorry." For our purposes, however, what is crucial is how invocation of the precautionary principle has influenced the assessment of the available scientific evidence on highly visible questions regarding health and the environment. Statements justifying use of the principle imply that the available scientific evidence bearing on a question will be evaluated in a rigorous and unbiased manner. In practice, a reflex emphasis on precaution can often favor poor science that appears to point to a risk and ignore higher-quality science that, if appreciated, would allay fears. Too often invocation of the precautionary principle avoids the challenge of critically evaluating the scientific evidence, making judgments about the magnitude and probability of a risk, and balancing costs and benefits. Too often it amounts to a rhetorical device, which is used to arouse the public on a particular issue. The assumption that the science will be judged on its merits is hard to maintain when there are numerous examples of influential organizations issuing assessments that favor positive findings over null findings and ignore the distinction between "hazard" and "risk" (see above).[26]

## CONTROVERSIES CONCERNING ENVIRONMENTAL HEALTH

Scientists routinely disagree in their assessment of the evidence on a given question, and questions pertaining to environmental, lifestyle, and dietary factors that may affect health are particularly subject to controversy. As we have seen, studies on these questions tend to have serious limitations, and scientists can have a strong investment in their work that goes beyond the science. As a result, what often characterizes these disputes is the intense attachment of some researchers to a given position—often based on favoring the evidence from particular studies that appear to show positive results. But it is important to recognize that the two parties in disputes are not necessarily equal in standing. In some cases, scientists on one side of the issue will make a concerted effort to evaluate all the relevant evidence in order to make sense of anomalous findings and come to a reasoned assessment based on the totality of the evidence. We will see examples of this when we discuss cell phone radiation and "endocrine disrupting chemicals."

In other cases, controversy on a topic of public health importance may be implicit, rather than being overtly acknowledged. For example, a recent evaluation of the controversy concerning salt intake and health documented a "strong polarization" in published studies.[27] Published reports on either side of the hypothesis—that salt reduction leads to public health benefits—were less likely to cite contradictory papers. Most striking was that, rather than acknowledging the existence of conflicting studies, the two camps tended to ignore each other and to be "divided into two silos." The tendency to ignore contradictory studies represents an abdication, since it is only by critically evaluating the relative merits of different studies and identifying the reasons for the conflicting conclusions that progress can be made. The authors pointed out that this pattern of researchers being divided into different camps, or "silos," characterizes other controversies, such as that concerning electronic cigarettes.

Needless to say, it would be very hard for the uninitiated to penetrate what is going on and to sort out the science from the rhetoric. And so disputes of this kind further confuse the public's understanding of the science.

## CONSENSUS

Compounding the many vexed issues surrounding questions relating to health and the environment is the simplistic notion that the "consensus among scientists" is always correct. This is a widely invoked criterion or shortcut for determining who is "right" in a scientific controversy. However, the results of a scientific study should not be expected to line up on one side or the other of a neat yes/no dichotomy. Unfortunately, the science is not always clear-cut, and the consensus on a particular question at any given moment may not be correct. Until the 1980s the consensus was that stress or eating spicy foods caused stomach ulcers. For roughly a decade, virologists believed that herpes simplex virus was the cause of cervical cancer. For more than three decades, the medical community believed that the use of hormone therapy by postmenopausal women protected against heart disease. The history of medical science is littered with long-held dogmas that, when confronted by better evidence, turned out to be wrong. We have to realize that appeals to the consensus are motivated by politics and have little to do with science. All it takes is for one or more scientists to come up with a better hypothesis and do the right experiment or make the right observation to overturn the reigning consensus.

* * *

This inventory of biases and tendencies affecting the interpretation and reporting of research findings is not exhaustive. Nevertheless, one can see that many of these tendencies can be at work simultaneously and can reinforce each other. This makes it easier to see how information cascades and bandwagon processes can get started. What is most surprising is that, as was said earlier, the items listed above are either axioms of research or pitfalls that are tacitly assumed to be guarded against by individual investigators and the scientific process as a whole. Thus it seems that there is a collective blind spot, and that in order continue to do these kinds of studies there is an unquestioned assumption that somehow, in spite of the well-known "threats to validity," informative research can still be carried out. Since we have examples of robust, transformative research findings, a crucial question is: how does one distinguish between research that is on a productive track and research that is focused on a problem that is unlikely to yield strong results or that, worse, is stuck in a blind alley? Why does work on certain questions get traction and make undreamed of strides, whereas work on other questions remains stalled?

Beyond the kinds of factors, principles, and tendencies described above that pertain to studies of health risks, to understand how certain interpretations and messages get imposed on the science, we need to step back and put science in the area of health studies in a framework that takes account of the psychological factors, professional circumstances, societal influences, incentives, pressures, fears, and agendas affecting what research gets done and how it gets interpreted and disseminated. For this purpose, work in the area of psychology and behavioral economics over the past four decades provides a crucial pillar of such a framework. Scholars in this area have produced seminal studies on errors in judgment, the perception of risk, and the mechanisms by which unfounded health scares can evolve and gain widespread acceptance, leading to misguided policies and counterproductive regulation.

## COGNITIVE SHORTCUTS AND BIASES:
## TWO SYSTEMS OF THOUGHT

In his book *Thinking, Fast and Slow* (2011), the psychologist Daniel Kahneman summarized decades of work with his colleague Amos Tversky on cognitive biases and pitfalls that affect judgment and to which we are all susceptible.[28] Kahneman distinguished between two different faculties of thought, which function according to very different rules. He referred to the two faculties as System I and System II. System I involves our automatic response to our environment and enables us to navigate our surroundings and to recognize many situations on the basis of stored experience without having to consciously analyze what is going on. It is System I that endowed our ancestors in the African savannah with the capacity to survive against omnipresent threats. This system is attuned to any possible danger and mobilizes the fight-or-flight response. If a hunter-gatherer heard a rustling in the grass, he had to decide instantaneously whether the sound signified the presence of a lion or merely the wind. In this situation, it made sense to react as if the rustling pointed to the presence of a lion, since the cost of being wrong was likely to be fatal. Even though the environment we live in is dramatically different from that of our forebears, System I has remained intact and is an integral part of our apparatus for interpreting the world. It is constantly at work, responding to cues from our surroundings, making split-second decisions, rendering judgments, which are generated below the level of our awareness. Most of the time System I serves us well and allows us to pay conscious attention to certain things, while carrying out many routine operations without consciously thinking about them. However, because it involves fast thinking, at times it can cause us to miss crucial information and make mistakes. System I is characterized by what feels right and natural. A compelling story, which engages us and confirms our expectations, will appeal to System I. It may be wrong, it may not be logical, and it may conflict with other things that we know, but if it is powerful and vivid and conforms to our deepest beliefs, it is likely to have a strong influence on our judgment.

In contrast to System I, the operation of System II, which acts on the inputs from System I, involves slow thinking. It can either endorse or rationalize the immediate thoughts and actions of System I or it can pause to take a slower, deliberate look at a situation. This latter course does not come naturally but rather involves reasoning, the weighing of possible outcomes, and judgments about future utility. Unlike the reflex responses produced by System I, Kahneman stresses that for System II to be able to correct errors made by System I requires continual vigilance and effort. And reasoning is an arduous process, in which our spontaneous reactions and feelings are of little help. All that matters is taking into account the relevant aspects of a choice or a situation and trying to decide what the outcome will be. Since System II requires effort and energy, we have a tendency to resist its demands and to slip back into accepting the judgments of System I. A key observation of Kahneman's is that, when we are confronted by a difficult question that demands serious thought, we often tend to substitute for it a simpler question to which we have a ready-made answer.

In a series of "thought experiments" carried out over many years, Kahneman and Tversky compiled an extensive inventory of cognitive errors that has transformed our understanding of everyday judgment and decision making. Such errors are the result of mental shortcuts, or "heuristics" (that is, rules of thumb) governed by System I, which work reasonably well in everyday life. However, especially when we are dealing with matters that are removed from our firsthand experience, they can lead to cognitive errors and biases. This is because our judgment is easily influenced by extraneous factors—our mood at a given moment, conspicuous information, vivid events that make an impression on us. All this happens below the level of our awareness.

The most fundamental shortcut that interacts with many other shortcuts to influence judgment is the *availability heuristic*, which is simply a mental shortcut or error whereby we judge the likelihood of an event by how easily we summon up instances of that event. The more "available" it is in our consciousness, the greater the importance we assign to it. For example, a recent, highly publicized crash of an airliner may affect our feelings about flying, even though we know that flying is far safer than other modes of transportation. Thus how easily we can summon up examples of a given event may bear little relation to its actual importance.

An appreciation of cognitive biases helps in understanding how distorted information regarding health risks can gain currency. The public relies on specialists to provide the interpretation of highly technical research findings. However, as we have seen, many results that are published are either tentative or wrong, and, furthermore, there is a strong bias toward positive results, even though these are likely to be false. Scientists are human, and their judgment in these difficult matters can be influenced by a variety of factors that have nothing to do with the strength of the science.

(Kahneman points out that even statisticians are susceptible to these kinds of errors.) Thus the difficulties and biases inherent in the conduct of studies in the area of health risks are embedded within an even more fundamental set of biases inherent in human behavior and society.

Although Ioannidis and Kahneman approach the question of sound judgment from very different perspectives—the one via statistical analysis, the other via the analysis of psychological processes operating at the most elementary cognitive level—these two bodies of work dovetail in unexpected and remarkable ways and provide a framework for understanding the confusion surrounding health risks. In both domains, there is a strong preference for positive results and coming up with a clear-cut and psychologically satisfying answer to a difficult question.

## AVAILABILITY CASCADES

Under the influence of the kinds of biases and shortcuts documented by behavioral psychologists, findings of scientific studies regarding threats to our health can gather momentum, becoming what Timur Kuran and Cass Sunstein have termed an *availability cascade*, or information cascade, or simply a bandwagon process.[29] This phenomenon is mediated by the availability heuristic, which interacts with social mechanisms to generate cascades "through which expressed perceptions trigger chains of individual responses that make these perceptions appear increasingly plausible through their rising availability in public discourse."[30] According to Kuran and Sunstein, this process comes into play in many social movements, as increasingly people respond to information from sources that appear to have some degree of authority. Information cascades can result in the mobilization of public opinion for positive ends, as in the civil rights movement and the spread of affirmative action. At other times, however, they can be triggered by "availability errors" (i.e., false information that gains prominence), and such cascades involving the mobilization of specific groups and the population at large can result in misguided policies or ill-conceived regulation.

Kuran and Sunstein's prime example of an availability cascade is the Love Canal incident of the mid-1970s, in which news reports concerning the contamination of a residential neighborhood in upstate New York by industrial chemicals snowballed into a national story, leading ultimately to federal legislation regarding Superfund sites. In this case, preliminary tests seemed to point to the existence of an imminent threat, and this alarming information was widely accepted and led to the evacuation of the neighborhood and compensation of homeowners. Only later, after years of more careful study by many scientists and agencies, did it turn out that, in fact, there was no evidence of any abnormal exposure among residents or any ill effects.[31]

The authors use the term *availability entrepreneurs* to refer to individuals or groups that play a major role in publicizing a risk or an issue and generating an availability cascade. In the Love Canal incident, an extremely vocal housewife played a key role in organizing homeowners and drawing media attention to the urgency of the health threat to the community. Responding to the community's concern, the New York State Department of Health declared a public health emergency, characterizing Love Canal as a "great and imminent peril."[32]

According to Kuran and Sunstein, availability entrepreneurs may believe what they are saying, or, more likely, they may be tailoring their public pronouncements to further a personal agenda, whether ideological, professional, philosophical, or moral. In the latter case, they are practicing what the authors term "preference falsification"[33] and others might call bad faith. If the results of a scientific study regarding a potential risk appear to conform to prevailing views in society, people will tend to accept the cited scientific findings as a result of this framing, even if the study reporting the result is weak. Those who question the solidity of the result or its importance on scientific grounds may be characterized as being "anti-environment" and "pro-industry," even when their skepticism is restricted to the evidence at hand. The concept of the availability heuristic helps explain how, as individuals and groups seek information about a given risk, the formulation of the issue by those with special knowledge can "cascade" through different groups and become solidified, becoming a widely accepted truth. One can easily see how these processes can have the effect of reinforcing the claim that the science is clear-cut and that a given risk is indeed a serious threat that we should pay attention to.

While a discussion of the role of scientists in the initiation and amplification of informational cascades is beyond the scope of their article, much of what Kuran and Sunstein say about availability entrepreneurs applies to scientists as well. Any account of the formation of public opinion on scientific questions must recognize that scientists are human and are social beings, as well as scientists. Their judgments about the importance of a given question can be influenced by factors that are extraneous to the science, including professional standing, the need to obtain funding, and moral and political beliefs. In other words, scientists themselves can be biased in their assessments and especially their public pronouncements regarding a particular hazard. This can lead to an emphasis on studies that show a positive association and ignoring studies that do not support the existence of a hazard. Scientists who act as availability entrepreneurs can count on the public's disposition to perceive their statements regarding an environmental threat as more trustworthy than statements that question the existence of a hazard.

## SCIENCE THAT APPEALS TO THE PUBLIC VERSUS SCIENCE THAT FOCUSES ON THE NEXT EXPERIMENT OR OBSERVATION

In this and the previous chapter, we have seen that findings from observational studies linking exposures to disease are only indications for further study and are not to be taken at face value. We have been badly misled by many intriguing findings that turned out to not be replicated when more careful studies were done. For this reason, the results of the "latest study" that get reported by the media have little claim to providing solid knowledge that is apt to make a difference in our life. To begin to be meaningful, the latest study needs to be seen in the context of all relevant work bearing on the question of interest. Most published findings turn out to be either wrong or overstated. Furthermore, the fact that a question is being studied is no guarantee that it is important or that a new hazard that has surfaced is something we need to worry about. Thus the assumptions implicit in much of the media reporting of studies in the area of health and disease are often directly at odds with the essence of the scientific process.

However, owing to the intense interest in anything that is possibly associated with our health, the perception of risks in the larger society can feed back on the science by giving undeserved support to certain lines of research and reinforcing certain fears or hopes.

\* \* \*

Science that deals with factors that affect our health takes place in a different context from other fields of science. This is because we are all eager for tangible progress in preventing and curing disease—a promise that is constantly reinforced by the media, medical journals, health and regulatory agencies, the pharmaceutical industry, and the health foods/health supplements industry. Until recently, medicine could do very little to treat or prevent most diseases, and people had a fatalistic attitude toward illness and death. But, with the enormous advances in biomedicine in the past fifty years, our desire for knowledge that will enable us to combat or stave off disease has become a distinguishing characteristic of modern society.

There are many urgent questions on which, in spite of an enormous investment of research funds and public interest, little progress has been made. We still do not understand what causes cancers of the breast, prostate, colorectum, pancreas, and brain, leukemia and lymphoma, Alzheimer's disease, Parkinson's disease, amyotrophic lateral sclerosis (ALS), scleroderma, autism, or many other conditions. Although we have learned a great deal about breast cancer over the past forty years, we still cannot predict who will develop the disease and who will not, and this applies to most other diseases. In contrast, there are other areas where dramatic progress has been made. These include the transformation of AIDS from a fatal disease to a manageable chronic condition; advances in the treatment of heart disease and breast cancer; the development of vaccines against human papillomavirus and hepatitis B virus—two major causes of cancer worldwide—and the identification of the bacterium that is responsible for most cases of stomach ulcer and stomach cancer. What this scorecard tells us is just how difficult it is to gain an understanding of these complex, multifactorial chronic diseases. The difficulty of making progress in answering urgent questions highlights the importance of identifying real issues and real problems by formulating new hypotheses and excluding possibilities by rigorous experimentation and observation.

* * *

In the following four chapters I examine two instances in which science has made dramatic progress in uncovering new knowledge that has translated into the ability to save lives and improve health (chapters 6 and 7) and two instances in which, in spite of abundant public attention, little progress has been made and little relevance to health has been demonstrated (chapters 4 and 5). By examining these two sharply contrasting outcomes of the research that attempts to identify factors that affect health, I hope to shed light on how, simultaneously, we expect too much and too little of science. Both sets of stories convey just how challenging it is to come up with good ideas and to make inroads into solving these problems.

Chapters 4 and 5 alert us to the waste and confusion that result from poorly specified hypotheses that generate bandwagon effects by promoting an unproductive line of research. Not all questions that are studied by scientists and receive both media coverage and funding are well-formulated or are based on strong prior evidence. And it is therefore not always surprising that, in spite of the hype, they do not lead to productive lines of discovery. (This does not mean that they may not merit study.) In fact, it is a reasonable working hypothesis that when a question is weak on purely scientific grounds but has salience for other reasons (such as its ability to inspire fear, or because it is associated with a political, ideological, or moral cause), this can compensate for its scientific weakness and can attract scientists, funding, and the interest of regulatory agencies and the public.

In contrast to such high-profile issues, there are other lines of investigation that have little resonance with the public but which, for purely scientific reasons, become the focus of sustained and rigorous, collaborative work that, over time, can yield results that could never have been foreseen at the outset. These represent productive veins of research, which prompt the development of new methods, the confirmation of results, and a deepening of understanding that can lead incrementally to important new knowledge. Where some instances of poorly defined research questions attract a huge amount of public attention, these other lines of research often do not relate to the common categories that evoke public interest and therefore tend to receive little media attention and to be confined to academic journals and professional meetings. They tend to get funded based on their scientific merit rather than on their appeal to the public. We can summarize this dichotomy by reversing Leo Tolstoy's formula about happy families in the opening sentence of *Anna Karenina*: "all poorly justified areas of study are alike; each truly important area of study is important in its own way."

This provides further support for the existence of a disjunction between "newsworthiness" and scientific value. It is easy to see why the latter stories don't have the same visceral appeal as the stories alerting us to a threat. Here we are talking about incremental steps, which may, in time, lead to a dramatic advances or even a breakthrough, but which don't stand out as starkly against the continuum of everyday life as the fears that erupt into the headlines.

\* \* \*

We can now see why certain questions that grab headlines and generate public concern have such enormous power and can take on a life of their own, casting a shadow over people's lives—remaining present in people's consciousness for a long period of time and, like a latent virus, being periodically reactivated by new stories that appear to point to the existence of a hazard. These scares appeal to our deep-seated instincts that react to a threat. Because the fear comes first—before a reasoned assessment of the evidence, which it bypasses—there is a sameness to the news reports that present evidence on the question. For this reason, the work that has addressed certain questions over a period of decades can appear essentially static. It never really gains traction, deepens, or evolves. Now this could be because the phenomenon under study is so weak as to be unimportant, and the hypothesis regarding its role in health or disease is wrong. Or it may be that the phenomenon is actually important, but researchers have not yet uncovered some crucial aspect of how it operates. In either case, the cause is not advanced by appeals to the public via the media, press releases, and health advisories. Progress can come only from the hard work of excluding alternative hypotheses and forging strong links in the chain of causation.

The demands of identifying and pursuing a productive line of research—one that eventually yields important new knowledge—leave no room for self-indulgent appeals to the public and solemn, self-serving warnings about the potential relevance of some unconfirmed, weak, and questionable finding to the public at large. As we will see in the two final case studies, the trajectory leading to major discoveries appears simple and straightforward only in hindsight. In reality, it is typically fraught with methodological obstacles, disputes between rival groups, efforts to improve methods, and uncertainty that the whole undertaking is really going to lead somewhere and not fall apart. For these reasons, in contrast to questions that invoke the specter of an insidious and imminent threat to our well-being, the stories that follow the tortuous "long and winding road" leading to a major discovery are not simple and have little visceral, emotional appeal.

My reason for contrasting two sets of stories with very different trajectories and very different outcomes is this. If we have in mind a model of what a true advance in the area of public health looks like, this might provide a much-needed reference point for judging the many sensationalized findings that get so much attention.

# 4

# Do Cell Phones Cause Brain Cancer?
## *A Tale of Two Sciences*

---

The safety of mobile telephones is a pressing question, now that the brains of nearly half the humans on the planet have become exposed within a short span of time to a physical agent to which their ancestors' genes could not have adapted.

—KENNETH ROTHMAN

---

The question of whether exposure to radiofrequency energy from cell phones is carcinogenic erupted into the public arena in 1993 when David Reynard, a resident of St. Petersburg, Florida, brought a lawsuit against a mobile phone manufacturer, alleging that his wife's fatal brain cancer had been caused by her using a cell phone, which she held on the same side of her head as that on which the cancer developed. Although he lost his suit, Reynard went on *Larry King Live*, voicing his certainty that his wife's cancer had been caused by her prolonged conversations on her cell phone and attracting widespread media attention. "She held it against her head, and she talked on it all the time," he explained.[1] Owing to the novelty of wireless technology that was poorly understood by the public and the fact that little is known about what causes brain cancers, this dramatic anecdote was to have an enormous impact.[2] Among the misunderstandings that circulated then and now and that inflame public concern is the notion that electromagnetic fields from mobile phones are "radiation," namely, ionizing radiation, like X-rays and gamma rays. Health and scientific agencies know that electromagnetic fields from mobile phones are non-ionizing and so are distinctly different from ionizing radiation sources.

Within a week of the broadcast a congressional hearing was held urging the federal government and the wireless industry to undertake studies to examine the health effects of cell phone radiofrequency emissions. The National Cancer Institute was already engaged in studying the causes of brain cancer, and researchers there added questions regarding cell phone use to their questionnaire. The Cellular Telecommunications Industry Association set up a $27 million project to examine the health effects of cell phone use.

Several early studies appeared between 1996 and 2001 showing little indication of a link between use of cellular or mobile telephones and brain cancer, and these studies might have laid to rest concerns about hazards of the new technology. In fact, in an editorial in the *Journal of the National Cancer Institute* in 2001, the physicist Robert L. Park cited the failure of a large prospective study of Danish cell phone subscribers, along with basic biophysical considerations, as settling the issue.[3] A number of factors, however, were to ensure that the question of carcinogenic cell phones would remain in the public consciousness: First, use of cell phones was still limited, and the average duration of calls was low, but their use was expanding at a rapid pace, and the technology was undergoing change. Second, the fact that new studies were planned or in progress in many different countries assured that new results would be appearing and getting attention. Finally, the question of cell phones and cancer arose at the precise moment when fear of extremely low-frequency electromagnetic fields (EMFs) from power lines and electric motors and appliances was at its height,[4] and anxiety about these two forms of non-ionizing radiation shaded into each other.

By 2013 there were 300 million subscribers to cell phone service in the United States and nearly six billion subscribers worldwide. Commentators raised the possibility that availing ourselves of this incredibly useful—and now all but indispensable—technology could cause an "epidemic of brain cancer" in the future, and some characterized the expansion of wireless technology, with its unknown effects, as the greatest uncontrolled experiment ever conducted on human beings. Given the unprecedented uptake of this new technology, whose potential effects on health were poorly understood and difficult to study, many scientists and health officials voiced concern about possible consequences. As the epidemiologist Kenneth Rothman, who has been involved in studying the health effects of mobile phone use since the issue first arose in the mid-1990s, put it, "The safety of mobile telephones is a pressing question, now that the brains of nearly half the humans on the planet have become exposed within a short span of time to a physical agent to which their ancestors' genes could not have adapted."[5]

The question of cell phones and cancer provides a prime example of how what appears to be a purely scientific question can be influenced by factors that have little or nothing to do with science and by the reciprocal interactions between the scientific community—and even within subgroups of the scientific community—and the larger society, including the general public, special interest groups, and health and regulatory agencies. Perhaps the most important bias of all those discussed in the preceding chapter is that of pretending that "the science is the science" and can be insulated from the fears, misconceptions, and agendas that are set in motion by the publication of "scientific findings" and dramatic anecdotal reports, such as that of David Reynard. It is disingenuous of scientists in the field of public health to pretend that their research is not affected by, and does not have effects in, the wider public sphere. However, before examining the science—or, rather, different versions of science—relating to cell phones and brain cancer, we need to briefly examine the basic facts about the two phenomena that are being linked.

* * *

Tumors of the brain, which can be benign or malignant, are extremely rare. Each year in the United States there are approximately 13,000 new cases in men and 10,000 cases in women.[6] For comparison, there are roughly 230,000 new cases of prostate cancer and an equal number of breast cancer cases. Cancers of the brain account for 1.4 percent of all cancer. Little is known about what causes these cancers. The only established risk factors are, in fact, exposure to ionizing radiation and certain rare hereditary conditions, which account for only a small proportion of cases.

To understand what is meant by cell phone "radiation," we need to situate this type of emissions in the electromagnetic spectrum (fig. 4.1). Electromagnetic energy consists of electromagnetic waves that are oscillations of electric and magnetic fields that travel at the speed of light. Electromagnetic energy can be characterized by its frequency (the number of oscillations per second) or wavelength (the distance between the crests of two waves). The higher the frequency, the greater the energy carried by the waves and the shorter the wavelength. Thanks to quantum mechanics, we know that the energy of the waves comes in discrete packets called photons. A given total energy of lower-frequency waves is made up of many very low-energy photons. The energy of higher-frequency waves is made up of fewer higher-energy photons.

Electromagnetic energy exhibits an enormous range from gamma rays, which carry the highest-energy photons, to 60-Hertz waves from the

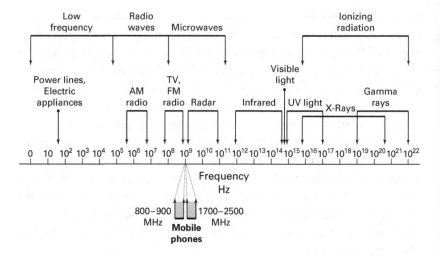

Figure 4.1
The electromagnetic spectrum.
*Source*: Adapted from Savitz and Ahlbom 2006. By permission of Oxford University Press.

electric power distribution system, which are made up of many very low-energy photons. Gamma rays and X-rays have very short wavelengths and very high photon energies, and for this reason they can damage molecules in our cells by "ionization"—that is, by knocking an electron out of an atom. The region of the spectrum that is involved in wireless telecommunications is in the kilohertz to gigahertz frequency range, spanning FM radio waves and microwaves. (For this reason, both terms are used in discussing the health effects of cellular telephones in the scientific literature.) This band of the spectrum is well below that of visible light and infrared energy, and the photon energies are far too weak to cause ionization. Microwaves can cause heating—as in microwave ovens—but only at much higher power levels than those used in wireless communications. In fact, the highest frequencies used in wireless communications, roughly 2000 MHz, are such that the photon energies are much smaller than the relevant biological energies.

A cell phone user's main source of exposure to radiofrequency energy comes through the antenna embedded in the phone, and his or her degree of exposure depends on a number of factors, including the characteristics of the phone and the distance of the antenna from the head; the greater the distance, the lower the exposure. Exposure is also influenced by the strength of the signal sent to the nearest base station, which is determined by how strong a signal the handset is receiving (i.e., the weaker the signal from the base station, the higher the exposure from the handset).[7]

The main effect of microwaves on living organisms is heating. A number of other effects (not related to heating) have been demonstrated, but these require high exposure levels. Standards for exposure to RF and microwave fields for workers and the general population have been in existence for decades, and these are based on microwaves' ability to heat tissues by transferring energy to molecules. The rate at which energy is absorbed by human tissues is measured by the specific absorption rate (SAR), and it is this value that is regulated to limit a cell phone user's exposure. In the United States, the Federal Communications Commission (FCC) has adopted the standard of 1.6 watts per kilogram, averaged over 1 gram of tissue for the head, recommended by the Institute of Electrical and Electronic Engineers. In Europe, the limit is 2 watts per kilogram averaged over 10 grams of tissue set by the International Commission on Non-Ionizing Radiation Protection (ICNIRP). These standards are conservative, providing a margin of safety that takes into account "worst-case scenarios." The underlying assumption is that with an adequate safety margin below the level at which microwaves can heat tissues, the likelihood of adverse biological effects is essentially zero.

Still, questions remain about the impact of exposure to RF on human tissues. One of these is the concern, voiced by some, that the limit for the amount of RF energy set by the FCC is based on the dimensions of an average adult male and therefore may be inadequate to protect women and particularly children, whose heads are smaller. Another area of concern stems from extensive laboratory studies that attempt to gauge the effects of RF exposure on cells and test animals. These studies are difficult to perform, and the aspects of exposure that are most relevant are unknown.[8] In this situation, there have been many claimed effects, and concerned groups have seized on these as evidence that RF may indeed be subjecting cell phone users to imperceptible damage that could lead to cancer or other diseases.

\* \* \*

Following the publication of several early studies, new epidemiologic studies continued to come out, primarily in Europe and the United States, and these continued to keep the issue in the public eye and to elicit divergent readings from scientists and interested parties. It has been the epidemiologic studies that have received the most attention in the media as well as in the health and regulatory community, and therefore it is important to examine what these studies entail and why it is so challenging to obtain clear-cut results regarding the possible association of cell phone use with brain tumors.

First, as mentioned earlier, brain tumors and tumors of the head are exceedingly rare, and specific types are even rarer, which makes them hard to study. The most common types of tumors of the brain and head are glioma (a malignant cancer), meningioma (usually a benign tumor of the membrane surrounding the brain), and tumors of the acoustic nerve (almost all benign) and the salivary and parotid glands (mostly malignant). Because of the rarity of brain tumors, the most common type of study used in their investigation is the case-control study, in which cases with the disease and controls (often selected from the general population) are interviewed to obtain information, and the two groups are then compared to identify differences that may be relevant to the development of the disease. The other type of study design that has been used to study brain tumors, but less frequently, is the cohort study, in which information is collected from a large, defined group of healthy individuals who are then followed for a number of years to monitor the development of disease. The exposures of cohort members who develop brain tumors can then be compared to those of cohort members who did not develop the disease. For a rare outcome like brain tumors, however, very large cohorts need to be assembled and followed, and this is very costly and time-consuming.

Although the case-control approach is more practical, this type of study has serious drawbacks. Because the desired information about exposure is obtained after diagnosis of the cases, this information can be affected by the presence of disease—for two distinct reasons. Cases with a serious and often fatal brain tumor may ruminate about what led them to develop their illness and may answer questions differently from healthy controls. Moreover, the brain tumor itself may affect the cases' cognition and memory. This difference between cases and controls in answering questions—which is independent of their actual exposures—is referred to as "recall bias" and can produce spurious results. In addition, since many brain tumors are fatal, some patients will die before they are able to participate in the study, resulting in a possible unrepresentativeness of the cases who are included.

But the greatest problem confronting both types of studies (case-control and cohort) is that of accurately assessing an individual's exposure to radiofrequency energy. To date, epidemiologic studies have relied on rather crude proxies for actual exposure.[9] Typically, study participants in a case-control study are asked questions about when they first used a mobile phone, how many calls they make and receive each day or week, how many minutes they usually talk on the phone per day, and on which side of the head they usually hold the phone, if they have a preference.

This requires respondents to recall their usage pattern going back as much as a decade or more. But usage patterns may have changed, and recall may be faulty. Moreover, people can hold the device in different ways that may affect their exposure, and they may have used hands-free attachments for some portion of their usage history. Another strategy that has been used in cohort studies has been to use billing records of mobile phone subscribers to estimate usage. While this approach avoids the problem of recall bias, it has other limitations as a measure of RF exposure (e.g., billing records may not capture actual exposure).

Another complication is that cellular technology has continued to develop rapidly over the past twenty years and has gone through four generations, including analog, digital, and digital UMTS. This further complicates the assessment of an individual's exposure over time.

Finally, brain tumors can take several decades to develop. But cell phones have only been widely used for the past ten to fifteen years. This means that not enough time has elapsed to gauge the full effects, if any, of exposure to RF. What we really would like to know is the effect of lifetime use of these devices, starting at an early age and at current levels of use (which for some people can amount to hours per day). Most currently available studies provide information on only a relatively short duration of use, at generally lower levels, and to earlier generations of cell phones.

These points are crucial to bear in mind when interpreting the results of studies conducted to date, and so their interpretation and the weight of different considerations requires care and an awareness of their substantial limitations.

As mentioned earlier, the timing of this new "radiation" hazard was significant in that it arose at the height of the furor surrounding the possibility that extremely low-frequency electromagnetic fields from power lines and electric appliances posed a threat of childhood leukemia, brain tumors, and other cancers. Many scientific studies of EMFs were in progress at that time (in the 1990s), and both the federal government and the electric power industry had programs devoted to research and education in this area. The media reported the results of each new study that seemed to hint that exposure to EMFs was associated with an ever-growing list of diseases—various types of cancer, heart disease, depression, Alzheimer's, Parkinson's disease, miscarriage, and so on. It was common to have scientists interviewed on the nightly news about the results of the latest study, with the ominous image of high-voltage transmission lines as the backdrop. Within a few years, as better studies were published, the notion of a threat from EMF exposure to the general population lost support in the scientific community.[10]

The fear instilled in the public was longer-lived, however, and the focus on this new form of non-ionizing radiation—radiofrequency fields—picked up where EMFs had left off.

\* \* \*

New studies continued to come out in the first decade of the new millennium. A number of these were part of a large and ambitious collaborative project, which was conceived in the late 1990s, when several groups of scientists recommended that the International Agency for Research on Cancer, an arm of the World Health Organization, investigate the relationship between cell phone use and brain tumors. After conducting a feasibility study, the agency determined that a multicountry case-control study would be both feasible and informative. The resulting INTERPHONE study was a population-based case-control study carried out in thirteen countries (four Scandinavian countries, France, Germany, Italy, the United Kingdom, Australia, New Zealand, Canada, Israel, and Japan), using a common protocol. The study focused on cases of brain tumors occurring in younger people, 30–59 years of age, since this group was expected to have the highest prevalence of cell phone use in the previous five to ten years.[11] The four tumor types included in the study were those occurring in tissues most likely to absorb RF energy emitted by cell phones: tumors of the brain (glioma and meningioma), acoustic nerve, and parotid gland. The data collection phase of the study ran from 2000 to 2004.

The results from a number of individual countries or groups of countries participating in INTERPHONE were published in the 2000s, and these gave some insight into the overall study results. It was not until May 2010, however, that the combined results for all participating countries were finally published. To appreciate the significance of the results when they finally came out, it is important to describe views on the question of cell phones and brain tumors held by both scientists and advocates who were to articulate the messages that influenced the regulatory as well as the public discussion.

By 2009 nearly thirty studies of cell phone use and risk of various tumors of the brain and head had been published. A critical assessment of this body of evidence by the Standing Committee on Epidemiology of the International Commission for Non-Ionizing Radiation Protection (ICNIRP) concluded that:

> Overall the studies published to date do not demonstrate an increased risk with approximately 10 years of use for any tumor of the brain or

any other head tumor. Despite the methodologic shortcomings and the limited data on long latency and long-term use, the available data do not suggest a causal association between mobile phone use and fast-growing tumors such as malignant glioma in adults (at least for tumors with short induction periods). For slow-growing tumors such as meningioma and acoustic neuroma, as well as for glioma among long-term users, the absence of association reported thus far is less conclusive because the observation period has been too short.[12]

This paper, written by a number of epidemiologists who have been involved in research on the health effects of non-ionizing radiation for decades, is noteworthy for its thoroughness and clarity. It attempts to provide an impartial summation of the human evidence, acknowledging the many limitations and potential biases inherent in the studies but at the same time providing some measure of reassurance, owing to the lack of any strong or consistent signal indicating a carcinogenic hazard. For this reason, the ICNIRP assessment stands in contrast to what has been made of epidemiologic and other data relating to cell phones by a small but vocal group of advocates, including some scientists, who take a very different view of the cell phone issue and who have had a disproportionate influence on the tone of the public discussion. The view articulated by ICNIRP in periodically updated publications is embraced by the majority of mainstream cancer epidemiologists and is in agreement with assessments by other groups.[13]

Studies from one group of investigators, led by the Swedish oncologist Lennart Hardell, stand out from the majority of studies and have been referred to as "outliers" or as discordant in a number of critical assessments of the overall evidence.[14] Starting in 1999, Hardell and colleagues published a series of studies that appear to show evidence of an increased risk of certain tumor types among long-term users of mobile phones. For example, in a paper published in 2006, these researchers reported that users of digital cell phones had a near doubling of risk of glioma (odds ratio 1.9) and that long-term users had more than a threefold increased risk (odds ratio 3.6). In more recent publications, Hardell and colleagues have reported that tumor risk was increased on the side on which was cell phone was held, and Hardell has declared RF energy to be a known carcinogen. However, cautious interpretation of these results is warranted for a number of reasons. First, as is the case for all case-control studies, there is concern about possible recall bias (that is, that cases with brain tumors may recall their past use differently from "controls," and that they may emphasize their exposure in order to account for why they developed their illness). It is also noteworthy that in the 2006 report even "short-term" users of digital cell phones (those who reported using them for one to five years) showed evidence of an increased risk (odds ratio 1.6). As we will see shortly, this result is at variance with the results of the much larger INTERPHONE study, as well as with the results of other studies from Sweden. Furthermore, it has been pointed out that, if such short duration of use were associated with brain cancer, this would be apparent in nationwide Swedish cancer rates after 2002–03 (the years cases were diagnosed in the Hardell study).[15] In fact, Swedish brain tumor rates have shown no increase through 2009. And there are similar data for the United States and the Nordic countries as a whole.[16]

In addition, questions have been raised about the methodology of the Hardell studies. For example, although the researchers used mailed questionnaires to obtain information from cases and controls, they reported participation rates of nearly 90 percent, which are highly unusual for studies using mailed surveys. Finally, the results reported by Hardell and colleagues contrast with those from almost all other studies (including cohort studies, where recall bias is not an issue). In the ICNIRP assessment from 2009 of epidemiologic studies, the authors pointed out that, if one analyzed the data on glioma omitting the Hardell studies, there was no evidence of an increased risk for either short-term or long-term use. Other recent overviews have made the same point.[17]

In spite of the questions surrounding the Hardell studies, activists have seized on his findings as confirming their conviction about the adverse effects of RF exposure. Starting in 2007 groups in the United States published a number of reports alerting the public to the possible dire effects of cell phones on human health. First to appear was the "BioInitiative Report," which declared that "existing public safety limits" on the radiation from phones and other wireless technologies are "inadequate."[18] Next, in the summer of 2008 the head of the University of Pittsburgh Cancer Institute, Dr. Ronald Herberman, issued an unusual alert to the school's faculty, staff, and students citing new, but unpublished, evidence that cell phone use causes brain cancer.[19] In the summer of 2009 two additional reports appeared: *Cell Phones and Brain Tumors—15 Reasons for Concern: Science, Spin and the Truth Behind Interphone* and a report from the Environmental Working Group entitled *Cell Phone Radiation: Science Review on Cancer Risks and Children's Health.*[20]

Two of these authoritative-appearing documents had as "endorsers" or "participants" diverse rosters of PhDs and MDs, and others, including neurosurgeons, general practitioners, politicians, lawyers, educators, and a firefighter.[21] Two of the documents were adorned with suggestive images adding to their scientific cachet—in one case, what looked like a radiological scan in vivid colors showing the radiation from a cell phone penetrating the brain; in another, assorted images of cell phone towers, high-voltage transmission lines, and zeros and ones projected on the back of a man's skull.[22]

The basic thrust of these reports was to argue that there is credible evidence that mobile phone use is associated with increased risk of brain cancer and nonmalignant tumors of the brain, then invoke the "precautionary principle" and counsel "prudent avoidance" to reduce one's risk, and particularly that of children.

To the lay reader, and even to many scientists and physicians who were not familiar with this subject, these reports were likely to appear to be serious and impartial assessments coming from independent-minded scientists concerned about the public's welfare. Their authors, we are given to believe, are speaking out in order to expose the flaws of industry-funded research and inadequate government regulation, and to expose the truth that is being suppressed by powerful interests. And, as they were intended to do, these alarming reports received widespread coverage in the media.

What the reports have in common, and what is most striking to anyone who is conversant with the scientific evidence concerning the health effects of cell phone use, is the highly selective and slanted presentation they give of the relevant evidence. While pointing to the findings of various studies as cause for alarm, the reports studiously avoid a number of crucial considerations that would help put the matter in perspective. In other words, their agenda involves something other than attempting to provide the kind of critical and demanding assessment of the totality of the relevant evidence that, as we saw in chapter 2, is the only way to arrive at a sound, if provisional, judgment about a public health issue.

In citing results from the epidemiologic studies, they fail to discuss the weaknesses and limitations of the studies in an impartial way. One element of such a discussion is to recognize that these limitations and biases could act in opposing directions—they could result in a failure to detect evidence of a real hazard, but they could also spuriously create the appearance of a hazard where none exists. One of the glaring symptoms of the activists' tendentious approach to the evidence is that they tend to pay attention only to the former possibility and not the latter.

It is less Hardell's results than his style of argumentation that calls into question his objectivity. He and his colleagues write as if their positive results are to be taken at face value, that is, as evidence of a risk. This reflects an uncritical approach to data from observational studies in general and from studies on the question of cell phone use and brain cancer in particular. Hardell and colleagues seem to fall into the trap of equating "association" with "causation." It appears that they are believers, and they marshal the evidence in a selective manner to support their belief. Given his aggressive advocacy, it is highly significant that Hardell was one of the "participants" involved in the "BioInitiative Report."

In addition to the overview by the ICNIRP group, two other meta-analyses on cell phones and brain tumors were published in 2009. One of these, by V. G. Khurana, Hardell, and colleagues, concluded that "the results indicate that using a cell phone for >10 years approximately doubles the risk of being diagnosed with a brain tumor on the same ("ipsilateral") side of the head as that preferred for cell phone use. . . . The authors conclude that there is adequate epidemiologic evidence to suggest a link between prolonged cell phone usage and the development of an ipsilateral brain tumor."[23] The ICNIRP report presents a table displaying similar results, but some of the studies included by Khurana/Hardell and ICNIRP differ, and the ICNIRP had refrained from presenting a pooled estimate of risk for ipsilateral glioma because it felt that the data showed evidence of recall bias. In other words, people with a brain tumor may be more likely to misreport the side on which they held the phone as the side on which the tumor occurred compared to healthy controls.

The second meta-analysis was performed by researchers from South Korea and from the University of California at Berkeley.[24] The senior author is Joel Moskowitz of the University of California at Berkeley, and I will refer to this as the Moskowitz paper. This paper represents a curious exercise. Without providing any rationale for their approach, the authors divided studies into those that used "blinding" (i.e., the interviewers and researchers did not know who was a brain tumor case and who was a control) and those that did not. In the latter group were fifteen studies by different research groups in the United States, Europe, Israel, and Japan; in the former group were eight studies, seven of which were by Hardell and colleagues. When the studies using blinding were analyzed as a group, they showed a statistically significant association between any use of mobile phones and the risk of brain tumor, whereas there was no association in the group of studies that did not use blinding. However, the authors never justified their use of blinding as the primary criterion to judge the quality of the studies, and it was never made clear how the absence of blinding would mask an association. In reality, the existence of blinding in the Hardell studies was due to the fact that they used mailed questionnaires to obtain information from participants, whereas in most other studies cases and controls were interviewed in person, making it difficult for the interviewer to be unaware of who was a case. The Moskowitz meta-analysis confirms the observation that the results of the studies by Hardell and colleagues differ from those of other studies, and, while it provides no insight into the reasons for this difference, its authors make the subjective claim that the Hardell studies are superior owing to their "low bias."

It turns out that the person who apparently motivated Ronald Herberman, the founding director of the University of Pittsburgh Cancer Institute, to issue his unusual and unprecedented alert to his staff and community was the cancer researcher, author, and activist Devra Davis, who at the time held a position at the university.[25] Davis has long been on the front lines of efforts to identify linkages between environmental exposures and cancer. In the 1990s she was instrumental in persuading the federal government to conduct a study to examine links between environmental exposures and breast cancer on Long Island—which in the end turned up no evidence of any association.[26] She has postulated a role for endocrine disruptors in explaining a wide range of phenomena, from effects on wildlife to a role in human breast cancer.[27] More recently she has been calling attention to the potential dangers of wireless RF and cell phones in interviews, newspaper columns, and a popular book: *Disconnect: The Truth About Cell Phone Radiation, What the Industry Has Done to Hide It, and How to Protect Your Family.*[28]

We need people who draw attention to potential health threats that have received inadequate attention. However, when advocates present themselves as scientists concerned about public health, one is entitled to expect an informed and critical consideration of all relevant evidence. The danger lies in latching on to certain findings that appear to signal the presence of a hazard, while ignoring the totality of the evidence and, equally important, the limitations of the types of studies being cited. Reading the publications of Davis and other cell phone activists provides a textbook exhibit of giving weight only to positive findings because these appear most convincing to people with a strong belief that there is something going on to which regulators and scientists need to pay attention. In this mindset, every elevated risk estimate becomes a signifier of a danger that is being denied by those who take a more critical view.

A few examples from Davis's *Huffington Post* article (2010) will show what I mean. In the second sentence, she writes, "This thirteen country report found what every study that has ever examined people who have used phones for a decades [*sic*] or more has determined—top users of cell phones had a doubled risk of malignant tumors of the brain." Only that is not what the INTERPHONE study reported. Rather than Davis's "doubling"—which corresponds to a 100 percent increase—INTERPHONE actually reported a 40 percent increase in the risk of glioma among long-term users with the greatest cumulative number of hours (odds ratio 1.40, 95% confidence interval 1.03–1.89) (table 2). Davis's reference to a doubling of risk refers to a subanalysis, which partitioned the data by whether the cases reported using their cell phone on the same side as the tumor or on the opposite side (table 5). There, the risk of glioma among "ispilateral" phone users with the highest cumulative call time is doubled, whereas the risk of glioma among "contralateral" users with the greatest call time shows a 25 percent increase (which is not statistically significant). This is just one example of selecting a particular result that supports one's position, rather than accurately describing the full results. Furthermore, while Davis points to this result as unproblematic evidence, the ICNIRP report cautioned against putting weight on the risk for ipsilateral phone use because of indications that recall of "laterality" of phone use is biased. Davis goes on to cite the work of Moskowitz—again, incorrectly—and to refer to Hardell's work ("regarded as some of the best efforts in the world on this challenging topic"), which, she tells us, "concur with the INTERPHONE and Moskowitz results." We have just seen that Hardell's results do not in fact "concur" with the INTERPHONE results. As for the agreement with Moskowitz, only the results for the "superior" (i.e., blinded) studies "concur," and this is hardly surprising since they are based, with one exception, on studies by Hardell!

Another key component of the argument put forward by Hardell, Davis, Moskowitz, and others is, as Davis puts it, "that there is a growing experimental literature showing that pulsed micro-wave like radiation from modern cell phones disrupts living cells and causes our DNA to become unstable—signs of cancer and other chronic disease."[29] The problem here—and one that the believers and activists seem blissfully unaware of—is that these studies are extremely hard to do, and it is difficult to know what the relevance of their findings is to actual human exposure. Even more to the point, most studies in this area tend not to have been replicated by independent researchers—the single most important criterion for judging the reliability of scientific evidence. Thus breathless references to these kinds of studies reveal an inability or an unwillingness to assess evidence in a critical manner.

The reports by activist groups invariably invoke the precautionary principle to clinch their argument that there is good reason to expect harm from use of cellular telephones. As was discussed earlier, while sounding eminently reasonable ("better safe than sorry"), the precautionary principle does not offer a clear guide to action.[30] Furthermore, when partisans seek to publicize a skewed version of the evidence, playing up certain findings and ignoring other crucial facts, invocation of the precautionary principle amounts to a rhetorical device to give their position a semblance of reasonableness to those who are unfamiliar with the real issues involved. (Another problem that is rarely acknowledged by those who invoke the precautionary principle is that there are risks associated with the status quo—not just with adopting some new technology or industrial process.)[31]

Finally, it is revealing that Hardell and associates involved in the "BioInitiative Report" chose to indict exposure not only to RF energy but also to the much lower frequency electromagnetic fields from power lines, electrical appliances, and other sources. Their reading of the evidence as of 2009—a full thirty years' worth—shows an ability to screen out vast amounts of research that was done that does not support their contention that exposure to EMFs is a cause of leukemia, breast cancer, and other diseases.[32] Reports like the BioInitiative document are really directed at people who are not acquainted with the extensive published literature, starting with the National Research Council report in 1997 and the large National Cancer Institute study in the same year on electromagnetic fields and childhood leukemia, which concluded that there was no persuasive evidence of an association. The activists' modus operandi is made clear in their treatment of the question of the health effects of EMFs. Basically, they ignore the most powerful studies and the most comprehensive assessments, and in the isolated studies they point to they avoid making the crucial distinction between association and causation (that is they show no awareness of the need for caution in interpreting the results of observational studies); but they readily accept, without hesitation, the results of any study that purports to provide evidence of an effect of EMFs. This same approach is taken with RF.

Rather than adopting a critical attitude toward evaluating the evidence from epidemiologic studies, and referring to basic considerations that should be part of any informed discussion of the issue, these self-proclaimed experts utilize a number of tactics to argue for the existence of a hazard and to attempt to undermine results that do not support their position. One of these is the recurring claim that studies of cell phones that are supported by the wireless communications industry are less likely to find an association with brain tumors than studies not supported by industry.[33] Like the arbitrary use of blinding as a criterion for rating the quality of studies, this is a red herring, because INTERPHONE was only partly funded from industry sources and, in any event, the study was run by IARC and was well insulated from any influence from the telecommunications industry. To imply that the results of this high-profile study could have been manipulated, when an army of respected scientists was intimately familiar with all aspects of the study, is preposterous and merely reveals the cynicism of the believers.

Perhaps what is most disturbing is how a small group of highly motivated activists can present a distorted picture of the evidence that can have wide influence. They are careful to use the trappings of "science" in order to impress people who have no background in this area and to appeal to people's unconscious fears about "radiation" and their insecurities about who is telling them the truth.

\* \* \*

The long-awaited results of the entire INTERPHONE study—the largest study to examine the link between cell phone use and tumors of the brain and other tumors of the head, which cost twenty-five million dollars—were finally published in May 2010 in the *International Journal of Epidemiology*, more than ten years after its initiation. It included 2,708 glioma and 2,409 meningioma cases and matched healthy controls. The ambitiousness and complexity of the INTERPHONE study is hinted at by the nearly three pages of acknowledgement of the individuals involved in referring patients and collecting information at multiple collaborating sites within each country. The paper's authors totaled forty-eight. But perhaps the most telling statistic, which is nowhere mentioned in the twenty-page article, is that it took over four years for the authors to agree on their interpretation of the data and approve a final draft. This conveys some indication of the difficulties of interpreting this type of data, reconciling different viewpoints, and reaching a consensus.[34]

Overall regular use of a mobile phone, as compared with nonuse, was associated with *reduced* risk of both glioma and meningioma, a result the authors attributed to possible bias. Long-term users (ten or more years) did not have an increased risk. However, in an analysis that divided cumulative call time into ten categories, those in the highest category had an odds ratio for glioma of 1.40 (95% confidence interval 1.03–1.89), meaning a 40 percent increased risk over nonregular users. The second highest category, though, showed one of the lowest risks. Thus there was no suggestion of a trend toward increasing risk with increasing cumulative call time. The odds ratio for meningioma was 1.15 (95% confidence interval 0.81–1.62), or a nonsignificant

15 percent increased risk. Having reported these findings, the researchers were quick to state that "biases and error prevent a causal interpretation."

The core message of the paper was thus an ambiguous one—that cell phone use did not appear to increase the risk of brain tumors overall, but that there was some suggestion that users with the greatest number of cumulative hours of use might have a slightly increased risk. The authors cautioned, however, that these positive results could be affected by a number of biases and could not be interpreted as evidence of a causal relationship. The paper received worldwide media coverage.[35] An editorial by two epidemiologists associated with IARC that accompanied the article in the journal pointed out that the conclusions of the article tolerated "diametrically opposed readings."[36]

The ambiguity of the INTERPHONE results allowed different groups to interpret the findings in conformity with their views. Three different positions are discernable. One group, including the members of ICNIRP, recognizes the problems with the study and fails to find any strong or clear-cut support for an association. While referring to what is known about RF energy, the ICNIRP authors take a balanced and reassuring view of the issue, while acknowledging the need for continued monitoring of brain tumor rates. A second group includes Hardell and scientists and activists aligned with him. This group finds confirmation of a risk in the few isolated blips in the results, which the INTERPHONE authors cautioned about taking at face value. The third, more difficult to characterize, group is composed of epidemiologists associated with IARC who organized the agency's assessment of cell phones and brain cancer. We will come to this group and their more complicated and ambiguous position shortly.

In view of the biases inherent in case-control studies of cell phone use, the results of a nationwide cohort study from Denmark assume particular importance. Launched in the late 1980s, this study included all Danes thirty-five years of age and older who were born in the country after 1925.[37] The population was divided into subscribers and nonsubscribers of mobile phones. Over 358,000 subscribers were followed for eighteen years, and brain tumors were identified through the Danish Cancer Registry. No association of cell phone use, or of long-term cell phone use (ten or more years), with brain tumors was observed in either men or women in this study.

\* \* \*

Up until now, I have largely focused on the epidemiologic studies and their interpretation by different groups. It is the epidemiology that receives the most attention and stirs up powerful emotions because these studies involve actual human beings with brain tumors and point to possible associations, which are easily interpreted as indicating causality. However, there is highly relevant evidence from other sources, which, because it doesn't have the same human interest, does not receive anywhere near the attention that is devoted to the results of epidemiologic studies, which tend to grab headlines. This is true not only of the media and the public; it is also true of some epidemiologists. Filling in these other components of the picture leads to a more scientifically informed view of the issue.

First, a crucial piece of evidence that would help to put the cell phone question in perspective is information about the rates of brain tumors and cancers over the past twenty to thirty years in different countries. Cell phone usage has increased at a geometric rate over the past twenty years in the United States (fig. 4.2). In contrast, brain tumor incidence increased during the late 1970s and 1980s, owing to improvements in screening, but has remained flat and even decreased in recent years.[38] Furthermore, when rates are broken down by age category, no increase is seen in younger age-groups, those with the heaviest cell phone usage. An analysis of long-term trends in glioma and meningioma incidence in four Scandinavian countries failed to detect any clear change between 1974 and 2003.[39] Similar results have been reported from other advanced countries.[40] A further analysis of glioma incidence trends in the United States between 1992 and 2008—a period during which cell phone use increased from close to 0 percent to almost 100 percent—concluded that the rates were not compatible even with the lowest risk estimate (odds ratio of 1.5) reported by Hardell after ten years of cell phone use.[41] While not enough time has elapsed to gauge the full effects of long-term cell phone use, nevertheless these statistics showing no change in the incidence/mortality from brain cancers in the face of a dramatic increase in mobile phone use provide some reassurance. The fact that there is no suggestion of an uptick in rates of brain cancer over a twenty-year period is important, since within twenty years of the increase in cigarette smoking in the United States following World War I, there was already a noticeable increase in rates of lung cancer in men. The extraordinary expansion of cell phones has occurred at an even greater rate.

Second, hundreds of experimental studies have been carried out to understand the effects of RF waves on animals and cells. The most informative of these studies are long-term experiments in which one group of test animals is exposed to RF energy of defined characteristics, and their "tumor yield" is compared to that of control animals, who were not exposed. One early study

A

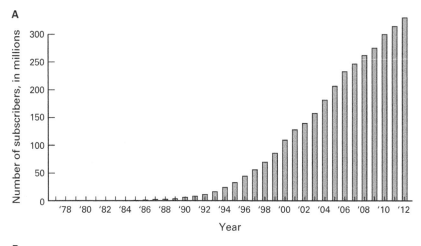

B

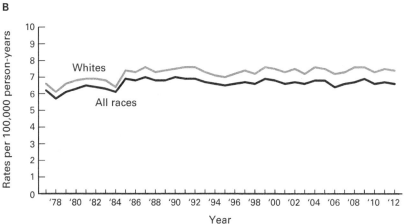

Figure 4.2
*A*. Number of wireless subscribers in the United States, 1984–2012. *B*. Age-adjusted incidence of brain cancer 1977–2012.
Adapted from Inskip, Hoover, Devesa 2010. *Sources*: Cellular Telephone Industry Association (CTIA). CTIA semiannual wireless industry survey 2012; SEER program, National Cancer Institute. By permission of Oxford University Press.

looked positive; however, the majority of studies show no evidence that RF of the type emitted by mobile phones is carcinogenic in laboratory rodents. In its 2015 comprehensive review of the health effects of non-ionizing radiation, the European Commission's Scientific Committee on Emerging and Newly Identified Health Risks (SCENIHR) concluded that these "well-performed," negative studies "provide strong evidence for the absence of an effect."[42]

Third, it is crucial to understand the properties of the agent in question, that is, the radiofrequency energy used in mobile phone technology. The first-generation mobile phones used frequencies in the 800 and 900 megahertz range, whereas the newer, digital technology uses frequencies in the 1800–1990 megahertz range. These frequencies are too low to induce or promote cancer by damaging DNA directly. While other "epigenetic" effects are theoretically possible, there is no reproducible evidence of such effects.[43]

One person who has attempted to put concerns about RF and electromagnetic fields in perspective is John Moulder, a professor of radiation oncology at the Medical College of Wisconsin, who has followed the research on these forms of energy for many years and produced assessments of the evidence. In 2005 he and his colleagues published a thoroughgoing, critical assessment of the evidence bearing on mobile phones and cancer. Their conclusions are worth quoting in full:

> Biophysical considerations indicate that there is little theoretical basis for anticipating that RF energy would have significant biological effects at the power levels used by modern mobile phones and their base station antennas. The epidemiological evidence for a causal association between cancer and RF energy is weak and limited. Animal studies have provided no consistent evidence that exposure to RF energy at non-thermal intensities causes or promotes cancer. Extensive *in vitro* studies have found no consistent evidence of genotoxic potential, but *in vitro* studies assessing the epigenetic potential of RF energy are limited. Overall, a weight-of-evidence evaluation shows that the current evidence for a causal association between cancer and exposure to RF energy is weak and unconvincing.[44]

Another figure who has attempted to understand the biophysical basis of possible health effects of RF and EMFs is Robert K. Adair, who is Sterling Professor Emeritus of physics at Yale University. Adair's career, spent at Yale and Brookhaven National Laboratory, had focused on high-energy physics, but in the early 1990s he turned his attention to the biophysics of the interaction between electromagnetic fields and biology. In 2003 he published an article entitled "Biophysical Limits on Athermal Effects of RF and Microwave Radiation" in the journal *Bioelectromagnetics*, in which he pointed out that there were no reproducible effects on biology of exposure to RF or microwave fields below the level at which heating occurs.[45] After considering a "complete set of possible biological interactions" involving possible athermal effects of low-intensity RF and microwave electromagnetic fields on human physiology, he concluded that it was "quite unlikely" that any mechanism could transfer energy exceeding the normal thermal noise of the human body. Hence he concluded that it is "most unlikely that RF or microwave fields of an intensity less than 10 mW/cm² incident on humans, can affect physiology significantly." But Adair went a step further. Referring to the eighteenth-century English mathematician Thomas Bayes, he argued that, when gauging the probability of an effect, one needs to take into account prior knowledge bearing on its likelihood. This is a much more sophisticated approach than simply examining each new finding in isolation, as if there were no previous relevant knowledge. Pointing to the body of published experimental findings purporting to show physiological effects of low-intensity fields, Adair commented that, given the theoretical implausibility of such effects, the results would have to be "especially definitive," since "remarkable conclusions—which seem to violate well considered principles—require remarkably strong evidence." In his judgment, the existing studies do not meet this standard. Note that Adair is not saying that it is impossible that RF could cause cancer. He is merely saying that, given everything that we know, it is extremely unlikely.

Although one cannot prove a noneffect, taken together, the results of the epidemiologic studies, the trends over time in incidence and mortality rates for brain tumors in many different countries, experimental evidence from studies in animals, and the biophysical considerations all converge in suggesting that cell phone RF is not carcinogenic.

\* \* \*

Since publication of the INTERPHONE results, several developments have helped to keep the question of the health effects of cell phone use alive and to deepen the confusion surrounding the issue. In February 2011 scientists at the National Institute on Drug Abuse and Brookhaven National Laboratory, led by Dr. Nora Volkow, published a paper in the *Journal of the American Medical Association* describing an experiment in which forty-seven volunteers, with a cell phone attached to both ears, were exposed to RF (without knowing which phone was activated), and glucose metabolism in the brain was measured.[46] The researchers found increased glucose metabolism—an indication of increased brain activity—in the area of the brain close to the antenna of the activated cell phone. The study received front-page news coverage and was seized on by many parties as demonstrating that RF radiation had a measurable effect on the brain. However, serious flaws in the design and interpretation of this experiment have been identified,[47] and in another study the effect went in the opposite direction—that is, glucose metabolism was reduced by exposure to cell phone energy. [48]

Then in May 2011 the IARC Working Group on cell phones and brain cancer issued a report declaring that radiofrequency energy from cell phones was "possibly carcinogenic."[49] Coming only a year after publication of the results of the INTERPHONE study, which showed no convincing evidence of a hazard, IARC's announcement left the public as well as many scientists nonplussed.

IARC is a prestigious agency that since the early 1970s has been producing respected monographs evaluating the evidence for a wide range of chemical, physical, and hormonal agents in the carcinogenic process. Later in this book we will see the important role played by IARC in identifying human papillomavirus as the cause of cervical cancer. However, in recent years several of the agency's assessments have been questioned on the grounds that IARC ignores real-world exposure and overemphasizes positive findings.[50]

What accounts for how IARC could evaluate all the relevant scientific evidence and come to an ambiguous conclusion, which meant one thing to scientists and quite another to a public concerned about the possibility of dire effects from talking on a cell phone?

IARC evaluates all available evidence bearing on whether a given compound causes cancer, including animal experiments, laboratory (mechanistic) studies, and human (epidemiologic) studies. However, as the agency makes clear in its preamble, it focuses on "hazard"—that is, any potential indication of harm, no matter how tenuous or under what artificial conditions—rather than "risk"—that is, the likelihood that significant exposure in real-world situations increases cancer in humans.

In addition to the agency's ignoring of the distinction between "hazard" and "risk," a number of irregularities in the committee's decision process regarding RF appear to have contributed to its baffling conclusion. The working group included Lennart Hardell, whose studies stood out from other epidemiologic studies in suggesting the existence of a risk. Two other epidemiologists on the committee resigned, one over an alleged "conflict of interest" and the other apparently in disgust at the proceedings.

Furthermore, although IARC routinely takes into account positive evidence of carcinogenicity from animal studies in its assessments, in the case of RF, panel members were instructed to restrict their attention to the epidemiology, thereby ignoring the high-quality, long-term animal experimental evidence that did not support a risk.[51]

The combined effect of these decisions was to give undue weight to the questionable findings of Hardell, who, in a clear conflict of interest, was voting on his own results.

All this raises the question: why did IARC have to carry out another exhaustive evaluation of the evidence? And once having carried out such a review, by any set of criteria for evaluating evidence, the conclusion should have been that, although we have not monitored the effects of cell phone use for long enough, the substantial evidence currently available provides no suggestion that cell phone use increases the risk of brain tumors. The Talmudic label "possible carcinogen" is unfortunate because it means one thing to scientists working for IARC and something quite different to the general public when trumpeted in the headlines.[52]

In classifying RF as a "possible carcinogen," IARC aligned itself with the precautionary principle, which sounds perfectly reasonable, except that it is often used conjure up the existence of a possible threat in the face of extensive and solid evidence suggesting the nonexistence of a threat.

We rely on health and regulatory agencies to provide impartial assessments of potential health risks. Unfortunately, the IARC cell phones report demonstrates that these institutions can be subject to the same political and professional pressures at work in society generally. The IARC review and the scientists who led it represent a third position intermediate between ICNIRP and the Hardell group. IARC straddles both camps and seeks to enhance its position by keeping the door open to a causal interpretation of very problematic epidemiologic data, but in its attempt to straddle both positions, it falls into incoherence, illogic, and ambiguity.

Rather than sticking to the science relevant to assessing a carcinogenic risk from cell phone use—which is IARC's stated mission—and reaching a conclusion along the lines of ICNIRP and SCENIHR, bowing to public opinion, the agency chose to venture into the territory of "risk management."[53] It succumbed to the temptation to convey a public health message rather than make a more boring statement about what we know. In doing so, it has confused the issue, since, if there is no convincing evidence of a risk, there is no compelling case for setting policy and alarming people unnecessarily. By its actions, IARC has only added to the confusion, since, as could have been expected, the public interpreted the "possible carcinogen" classification differently from the committee, that is, that cell phones can cause brain cancer. As the statistician Donald Berry is quoted as saying in response to the IARC announcement: "Anything is a possible carcinogen. This is not something I worry about and it will not in any way change how I use my cellphone," he said—speaking from his cellphone.[54]

\* \* \*

There seems to be a paradox—or rather, a number of interlocking paradoxes—at the heart of epidemiologic research examining the health effects of cell phone use. In this day and age, such studies are going to be done, and new studies of the cell phone question are in progress.[55] Given the existence of the field of epidemiology, the widespread and high-stakes concern about the potential carcinogenicity of radiofrequency energy, and the fact that evidence from human studies is considered the most relevant and valuable information for health risk assessment, agencies like the Environmental Protection Agency, the Food and Drug Administration, and the International Agency for Research on Cancer see it as their responsibility to consider these studies. Once studies are done, it goes without saying that the media will report their results. But even more important, once the results are published—once they are out there—those people disposed to find evidence of an effect will seize on certain results, even when extreme caution is in order in interpreting them. On the other hand, when evaluated critically by scientists with no axe to grind, the severely limited ability of these studies to answer the ultimate question they are designed to answer comes clearly into focus. In the worst case, studies like INTERPHONE can appear to be what the literary theorist Stanley Fish called "self-consuming artifacts." A rigorous and honest assessment of their limitations and potential biases can completely undercut the credibility of their results. And yet the one thing that is certain is that new studies will be undertaken. The problem with research in this area is not that it is worthless, but that all too frequently it is interpreted naively and uncritically and used for partisan rather than scientific purposes.

Given this situation, how are we to think about the possibility that cell phone use might cause brain tumors—when the issues involved are highly technical, involving radiation biology, epidemiology, and statistics; when a steady stream of studies has come out over the years showing what appear to be weak and conflicting results; and when the viewpoints of those who opine on this question are often dramatically at odds? If one steps back and tries to look at the attention devoted to this question in its totality—including the science that has been done, the interpretation of the science by different groups, the calls for more stringent limits on exposure; the legal challenges alleging harm due to cell phones; and, above all, the type of arguments that are made—one sees that certain crucial facts rarely get articulated in the public discussion, and this allows a certain type of rhetoric and weak logic to dominate. Even some of the most sophisticated commentators can have their field of vision narrowed and neglect to mention important considerations or can place undue weight on questionable findings.

One cannot understand a phenomenon like the anxiety surrounding cell phones without considering the social context in which "scientific" messages are disseminated. No matter how temperate and judicious scientists are in reporting their results, certain messages are much more likely to be received by the public than others, and we well know that the slightest statistical blip in the data can get translated as alarming evidence of an effect. A second, and related, point is that the quality of the science—and the sheer difficulty of conducting informative studies on certain topics—is rarely conveyed to the public. Of course, this is nowhere near as newsworthy or as titillating as the latest evidence that a new type of tumor or other illness has been linked to cell phone use. Third, while the results of epidemiologic studies involving the "outcome" of interest, namely, brain tumors in humans, receive a great deal of attention, relevant findings from other scientific disciplines tend to be ignored as being irrelevant or overly theoretical or esoteric, even by some of the most sophisticated people involved in assessing the health effects of cell phones. This conveys the erroneous message that the results of epidemiologic studies, which involve real human beings with tumors, are of immediate relevance. All these factors create a situation in which the relevant information regarding the potential health effects of using cell phones gets badly skewed. Examining this question in its appropriate context can provide insight into how a health issue can get distorted and can take on a life of its own and persist for years in spite of persuasive scientific evidence that the much-dreaded adverse effects are unlikely and that we should focus our resources and attention on other problems.

\* \* \*

We have to remember that the whole question of cell phone use and brain cancer arose not because of some strong piece of clinical or epidemiologic evidence or because of a strong theoretical basis for positing that RF was likely to cause cancer. Rather, it arose as a result of a single, dramatic case, which appealed to a distraught husband's desire for an explanation of what caused his wife's fatal brain cancer. On its face, the striking occurrence of a brain tumor on the same side of the head as that on which a person habitually held a cell phone can appear to many people as a decisive demonstration of cause and effect. In reality, it reflects the influence of the kind of cognitive biases described by Daniel Kahneman, since the odds of developing a tumor on one side of the head versus the other are about even. By means of prime-time television and print media, this powerful meme created what Timur Kuran and Cass Sunstein have called an "availability cascade" that entrained scientists, activists, national and international health agencies, and the public. If the cell phone question arose out of a poignant instance of an all-too-human bias, its unfolding over the past twenty years has provided ample occasions for the play of bias in many forms and at many different levels in the interpretation of the results of scientific studies and the translation of these results to the public.

# 5

# Hormonal Confusion
## *The Contested Science of Endocrine Disruption*

At the present level of knowledge . . . the idea of endocrine disruption is still in the hypothetical realm, and the scientific and regulatory community is still polarized between believers and detractors.

—A. C. VIDAEFF AND L. E. SEVER

In 1992 the *British Medical Journal* published an article entitled "Evidence for Decreasing Quality of Semen During the Past 50 Years."[1] The authors, from the University of Copenhagen, reviewed sixty-one papers from a wide range of countries that reported on semen quality from 1938 to 1991. Although previous studies had raised the issue of a decline in semen quality in selected populations, the *BMJ* paper was the first to take a systematic approach by considering all published studies of men without a history of infertility. Their "meta-analysis" (that is, an averaging of the results of sixty-one individual studies) showed that average "sperm count" had declined globally from $113 \times 10^6$ to $66 \times 10^6$/milliliter, or by 42 percent, from 1940 to 1990. Ruling out methodological variation and selection bias as possible explanations, the authors judged that their results reflected a "true biological phenomenon." They went on to make two additional leaps, first, suggesting that the sperm count results might reflect a decline in male fertility—the male's ability to father a child—and second, linking the decline to an increase in testicular cancer and other male genitourinary abnormalities, including undescended testes and hypospadias, a birth defect in which the opening of the urethra is not at the tip of the penis.

In their opening sentence, the authors referred to increasing concern "about the impact of the environment on public health, including reproductive ability." They closed with the words, "Whether oestrogens or compounds with oestrogen-like activity or other environmental or endogenous factors damage testicular function remains to be determined."

Since 1992 the paper has been cited 2,707 times in the scientific literature, an astonishing number for a scientific paper, and has been widely reported in the media. It appeared at a critical moment of mounting concern about the possible effects of environmental pollution on wildlife and human health, including increasing cancer rates, and particularly breast cancer. A particular focus of concern was possible harmful effects of exposure to synthetic chemicals, including pesticides, like DDT, aldrin, and dieldrin; industrial pollutants, like polychlorinated biphenyls (PCBs), dioxins, and heavy metals; and compounds released by the burning of fossil fuels. The Danish paper, with its implication of a drastic decrease in male fertility—conjuring up a possible end to human procreation—appeared to add one more piece of evidence that supported the mounting concern that exposure to chemicals accumulating in the environment from industrial and agricultural practices was having a wide range of effects throughout the ecosystem and was threatening the most basic biological processes.

A number of observations over the preceding decades had galvanized ecologists, reproductive specialists, and epidemiologists.[2] For example, male alligators in Lake Apopka, Florida, had become feminized following exposure to pesticides released into the lake from runoff and effluent from a sewage treatment plant. Trout had disappeared from the Great Lakes, possibly as a result of exposure to dioxin-like pollutants from industrial runoff. Children whose mothers had consumed sport fish from the Great Lakes scored lower on intelligence tests at age seven compared to children whose mothers had not consumed fish from that source. The decrement was associated with prenatal exposure to PCBs, which were found at high levels in sport fish from the Great Lakes. The babies' in utero exposure, indicated by umbilical cord blood levels, showed a significant association with lower scores on a visual recognition test.[3]

But by far the most credible and significant finding concerning the potential effects of exposure to chemicals on development did not involve an environmental exposure at all. Rather, it was the result of what is referred to as a "natural experiment." Starting in the 1940s and continuing through the 1960s, pregnant women with a history of bleeding or of prior miscarriage were given the synthetic estrogen diethylstilbestrol (DES) to prevent miscarriage. It is estimated that during this period three million women were given DES in the United States. In 1971 Arthur Herbst, a gynecologist at Massachusetts General Hospital, and colleagues published a landmark paper in the *New England Journal of Medicine* reporting that daughters born to women who had been prescribed DES during pregnancy were at increased risk of developing an extraordinarily rare cancer, clear-cell adenocarcinoma of the vagina, when they reached maturity.[4] This demonstrated that DES taken by the mother during pregnancy could cross the placenta and affect the cells of the vagina of the developing fetus in ways that resulted in the development of cancer decades later. In the language of biologists, DES was a *transplacental carcinogen*. The discovery of the effects of DES therapy was to serve as a model for research into the effects of exposure to chemicals in the environment on development.[5]

Rachel Carson gave powerful expression to concern about the potential impact of exposure to environmental pollution on the ecosystem and on human health in her best seller *Silent Spring* (1992). The years following the Second World War saw an enormous expansion of industrial production and modern agriculture, with the introduction of thousands of new synthetic compounds, and, in response to increasing evidence of far-reaching impacts of these developments, a multifaceted environmental movement evolved throughout the 1960s and 1970s.[6] This new environmental consciousness led to the creation of the Environmental Protection Agency in 1970 and the enactment of the Clean Air and Clean Water Acts. Also in 1970, President Richard Nixon declared a "War on Cancer" and expanded the mission and responsibilities of the National Cancer Institute.

Another, rarely cited, factor that was to influence the new environmental awareness dates from the late 1960s, when influential epidemiologists posited that the vast majority of cancer was due to "environmental factors." The term "environment" was used in the broadest sense to include lifestyle exposures and behaviors, such as smoking, diet, alcohol consumption, infectious agents, and chemical exposures, as opposed to genetics. The public widely, if understandably, misunderstood this axiom to mean mainly exposure to pollution, including trace amounts of chemicals in the external environment.[7] This unfortunate misreading of the concept of the "environment" as it relates to the development of disease has been widespread and persistent and has been the source of much confusion surrounding the role of contaminants in food, air, and water and their contribution to disease.

Throughout the 1970s and 1980s interest in the possible impact of environmental pollution on disease focused overwhelmingly on cancer.

This focus was amply fueled by industrial accidents (Times Beach, Missouri; Seveso, Italy; Three Mile Island, Pennsylvania; Chernobyl, Soviet Union); the Love Canal incident in upstate New York; the identification of thousands of toxic waste sites and contaminated wells; reports of drinking water contaminated by low levels of chlorinated compounds and other industrial chemicals, pesticides, and oral contraceptives; and cancer clusters, like those in Toms River, New Jersey, and Woburn, Massachusetts.

This is where things stood in the early 1990s, when the many varied observations in wildlife and a number of apparent trends in human disease were to provide the basis for an ambitious and provocative new theory positing a linkage between a wide range of exposures and an equally wide range of health outcomes. The report concerning declining sperm counts was one example—although a prominent one—of the many possible impacts of environmental exposures that this new theory put on the agenda. The theory, known initially as the "environmental estrogen hypothesis" and later as the "endocrine disruption hypothesis," was formulated independently in the early 1990s on both sides of the Atlantic.

In the summer of 1991 a small group of scientists was brought together by Theo Colborn, a zoologist and ecologist who had spent years compiling data on the effects of environmental pollutants on wildlife and particularly documenting the effects of pollution of the Great Lakes. Meeting in Racine, Wisconsin, the group produced a consensus document, known as the "Wingspread statement," which highlighted the many findings underlying the hypothesis as well as its implications for human health.[8]  Under the heading "We Are Certain of the Following," the authors cited the extensive evidence regarding alterations in sexual development in wildlife associated with exposure to chemical pollutants in the environment, including decreased fertility, gross birth deformities, metabolic abnormalities, behavioral abnormalities, and changes in sexual characteristics. Many of these changes had been observed across a wide range of wildlife, including birds, fish, and mammals. The fact that some of these observations in wildlife appeared to be explained by biological mechanisms that had been identified in laboratory studies examining the effects of exposure to specific chemicals seemed to support a causal relationship.

A crucial aspect of the formulation was that the adverse effects of exposure could vary dramatically depending on the timing of exposure: whether this involved the embryo, the fetus, the newborn, or the adult. The effects, Colborn and colleagues noted, were most often manifested in the offspring rather than in the exposed parent. Thus exposure during embryonic development could result in birth defects but could also have delayed effects on reproductive ability, development, or metabolism that appeared only later in life. This was the import of the reported effects of in utero exposure to PCBs from contaminated fish on cognitive ability in children and, even more strikingly, of the DES experience.

To disseminate the endocrine disruption hypothesis to the widest possible audience, Colborn teamed up with a science writer and an environmental scientist to write the best-selling book *Our Stolen Future: Are We Threatening Our Fertility, Intelligence, and Survival? A Scientific Detective Story* (1996). The book carried a foreword written by then vice president Al Gore. By 1999 sixty-two thousand copies had been sold in the United States, and the book had been translated into sixteen languages.

Responding to the same body of seminal findings, scientists in Europe had independently formulated a version of the endocrine disruption hypothesis. They were aware of discussions in the United States on "estrogens and the environment" as well as the Wingspread statement. In 1993 Richard Sharpe of the University of Edinburgh and Niels Skakkebaek (the senior author on the paper showing declining sperm counts worldwide) wrote a hypothesis article in the *Lancet* that proposed that in utero exposure of males to estrogens (from various sources) might underlie common male reproductive disorders.[9] They vividly conjured up a possible role of xenoestrogens—that is, estrogenic compounds in the environment—pointing out that "humans now live in an environment that can be viewed as a virtual *sea of estrogens.*" In 2001 Skakkebaek formulated another variant of the endocrine disruption hypothesis, referred to as the "testicular dysgenesis syndrome hypothesis," which posited that fetal exposure to endocrine disrupting chemicals plays a role in malformations of the male reproductive organs, impaired sperm production, reduced androgen production, and testicular cancer.[10]

The endocrine disruption hypothesis articulated a new paradigm that was enormously successful in galvanizing the research community, environmental agencies, and the public to take seriously the hither-to neglected but potentially far-reaching and varied effects of environmental pollution on wildlife and human health. There had been a steady, low-level output of research papers on "environmental estrogens" from the late 1960s to the early 1990s, and these increased sharply in the early 1990s. The number of scientific publications on "environmental endocrine disruptors" listed in the National Library of Medicine's online bibliographic database surged from 4 in 1995 to 427 in 2013.[11] As scientific and regulatory attention to endocrine disruption grew, the topic began to receive regular coverage in the media. According to one observer, a review of print media mentioning endocrine disrupters revealed "the exponential rise of media attention to the issue from the early to mid-1990s."[12]

Responses to the hypothesis and its presentation in *Our Stolen Future* and in the scientific literature varied greatly. Without doubt, one of the more enthusiastic endorsements of the hypothesis came from Sheldon Krimsky, a scholar who focuses on science and public policy, in his book devoted to the endocrine disruption hypothesis, entitled *Hormonal Chaos* (2000). Krimsky called it a "bold and unorthodox hypothesis" that brought together results from different disciplines that no one had hitherto considered. He likened the potential importance of what he termed the "environmental endocrine hypothesis" to the discovery of chemical mutagenesis and the discovery that chlorofluorocarbons were depleting the protective ozone layer in the atmosphere.[13] In fact, Krimsky basically took Colborn and colleagues' own estimation of the hypothesis at face value. While the scientific community widely accepted the endocrine disruption hypothesis in a programmatic sense as defining an agenda for research, there were those who early on questioned some of the key assumptions behind the hypothesis or noted that the theory had little in the way of factual underpinnings.[14] Others appeared to accept the framework provided by the hypothesis—or rather, the bundle of questions subsumed under it—but never lost sight of the enormous difficulty of elucidating the effects of low-level environmental exposures on normal development.[15] Some scientists simultaneously carried out research studies but, at the same time, were severe critics of methodologically weak studies and one-sided claims.[16]

The success of the endocrine disruption hypothesis would depend on identifying an important contribution of a common, widespread exposure in the general population—or some substantial segment of the population—to the development of some disease or pathologic condition. For example, if it could be demonstrated that the increase in breast cancer, testicular cancer, male reproductive malformations such as cryptorchidism or hypospadias, or obesity was in a substantial way associated with, and preceded by, exposure to a particular chemical or group of chemicals in drinking water or food, or by other modes of exposure, and if removing or reducing this exposure led to a decrease in these conditions, this would provide solid and important evidence for the theory. After twenty years of research, regulatory attention, and abundant media coverage, it is reasonable to ask how the endocrine disruption hypothesis has fared, what new knowledge it has yielded, and what happens to science when it addresses a question that is both difficult to study and at the same time evokes powerful emotions and preconceptions. This chapter will examine what happened when research focused on specific disease trends and specific exposures to test the endocrine disruption hypothesis and how this research led to a tangled scientific and public controversy that shows no sign of abating. In view of the vast scope of the endocrine disruption hypothesis, I will confine my discussion to effects on human health, since the question of effects on wildlife involves different disciplines and different methods of study. Furthermore, it can be argued that the issues involved in these two aspects of the endocrine disruption hypothesis are so different that their conflation has contributed to the confusion surrounding the question of the effects of "endocrine disrupting chemicals" on humans.

* * *

Hormones are chemical messengers secreted by ductless glands and travel through the bloodstream to affect distant organs. Hormones play a crucial role in orchestrating the body's growth, maintaining physiologic balance, and sexual functioning and development. Estrogen and testosterone influence the development and the functioning of the reproductive organs; insulin regulates the body's level of blood sugar; thyroid hormones are important in regulating the metabolic rate. Hormones also orchestrate the development and functioning of many other tissues. The network of glands, hormones they produce, and receptors they bind to are collectively referred to as the endocrine system.[17]

Once secreted, a hormone must be transported via the bloodstream to the target organ by a carrier protein. Once there it binds to a receptor, and the hormone-receptor unit binds to a specific region of a cell's DNA to activate particular genes. Different synthetic compounds can influence hormonal activity in a number of ways. Some endocrine disruptors can mimic a natural hormone and bind to the hormone receptor, producing the same response as the natural hormone, or strengthening or weakening its effect. Other compounds can stimulate the production of more hormone receptors, thereby amplifying the effect. Still other compounds can block the action of a hormone simply by occupying the hormone's site on the receptor.[18]

A fundamental insight of the endocrine disruption hypothesis was that synthetic compounds such as the synthetic estrogen DES, pesticides including DDT, and industrial chemicals, such as bisphenol-A, could influence the body's hormonal pathways, even though their chemical structure

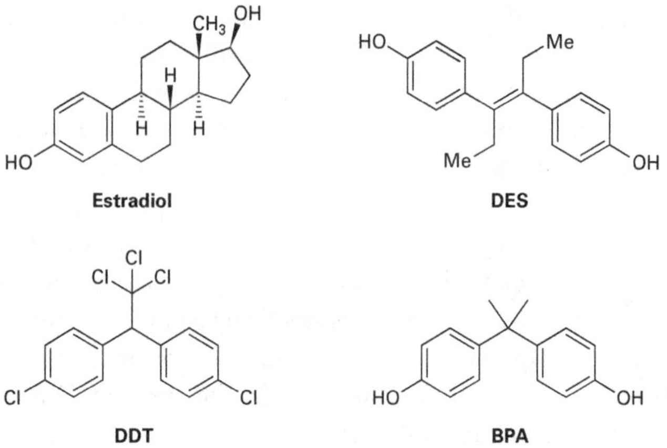

Figure 5.1
Chemical structures of several compounds with differing estrogenic potencies.
*Source*: Wikipedia Commons.

differed from that of the natural hormones estrogen and testosterone. The latter have a distinctive four-ring structure, whereas the former have a two-ring configuration (fig. 5.1).

The endocrine disruption hypothesis brought together a number of observations that raised the question whether exposure to chemicals in everyday life could be contributing to a wide variety of diseases and conditions, some of which appeared to be becoming more frequent. The scope of the hypothesis was vast, encompassing thousands of chemicals and a daunting number of different pathways and mechanisms—mostly unknown—by which these chemicals might affect biological development and functioning. Before discussing what has come of major lines of research on this question, I need to make some preliminary points that rarely get attention.

When considering the hormonal effects of different substances, it is crucial to keep in mind that estrogenic (and other hormonal) substances have different potencies, determined by their ability to bind to receptors and thereby elicit cellular responses. The hormonal effect of a substance will depend on its potency and concentration.

What research in this area demonstrates most vividly is how difficult it is to identify a specific causal factor when we are dealing with low- and very low-level environmental exposures in free-living populations. Much of what we know about the effects of exposure to chemicals comes from studies of occupationally exposed workers or from industrial accidents or accidental contamination of food or drinking water. Another source of information about the effects of exposure to chemicals comes from epidemiologic studies of exposures, including smoking, intake of alcoholic beverages, use of oral contraceptives, and postmenopausal hormone therapy, and studies of treatment with therapies like tamoxifen. We have solid knowledge about the effects of these exposures because they involve prolonged, habitual exposure (in the case of smoking and drinking) and relatively high levels of exposure (in the case of occupational exposures). When it comes to lower levels of exposure to contaminants in food, air, and water, the situation is very different.

First, any effects of such exposures may be subtle, transient, or nonexistent. Just because we can measure the presence of a compound in blood or urine using powerful modern technology does not mean that it is having a detectable effect. Second, lifestyle behaviors and exposures, such as smoking, drinking, diet, weight gain, physical activity, and breast-feeding, may overwhelm or modify any effects of environmental exposures. Third, an individual's genetic makeup is likely to influence his or her ability to metabolize and detoxify these exposures. Fourth, many environmental exposures involve mixtures rather than a single substance, and exposures are likely to change over time as a person's life circumstances change, making it difficult to obtain a complete record of exposure over the relevant decades. Finally, the types of studies that are done may be capable of picking up a strong effect, but if the effect is subtle or confined to a subgroup with particular vulnerability, few studies will have the ability to pick this up.

Beyond the difficulties inherent in establishing clear-cut effects of such environmental exposures on human health, there is a wider social context in which certain findings are disseminated and attract attention. And the existence of interested parties in the form of a concerned public, environmental advocates, the legal profession, government agencies, and scientists themselves can play a major role in how a scientific question is framed and perceived. When studies are done, they often appear to show an intriguing, novel, and important result, and such a result will inevitably generate excitement among researchers, who are looking for evidence of a relationship. Such results are also of great interest to regulatory agencies and, needless to say, the media. All too often, however, initial findings that appear to furnish evidence of an effect are not borne out when larger and more rigorous studies are carried out.[19] Moreover, it is basic reality that positive findings get more attention and, one could even say, are more psychologically satisfying and convincing than studies that find no effect. Such problems affect many areas of research into factors influencing our health, but when it comes to the endocrine disruption hypothesis, they appear—if one may put it this way—to be "on steroids."

* * *

From early on there were scientists who voiced skepticism regarding the endocrine disruption hypothesis. One of these was Stephen Safe, a toxicologist at Texas A&M University. In 1995 and again in 2000 he articulated a number of fundamental points that argued against exposure to industrially derived endocrine disrupting chemicals being responsible for a global decrease in sperm counts, decreased male reproductive capacity, or breast cancer in women.[20] Among his key points were the following. First, it is difficult to sort out causality in many of the alleged effects of environmental exposures on wildlife. In any event, the most striking instances of changes observed in wildlife were associated with unusually heavy exposure to pollution. Second, levels of exposure to synthetic estrogens in the environment are extremely low compared to concentrations of naturally occurring endocrine-active compounds in our diet (isoflavones). For example, according to Safe, levels of "estrogen equivalents" from organochlorine pesticides in food are on the order of one-thousandth that found in a standard portion of red wine or beans and closer to one-ten thousandth that found in cabbage. Third, alleged changes in male reproductive capacity are not correlated with differences in exposure to industrial pollution. Safe also pointed out that chemicals in the environment could have antiestrogenic as well as estrogenic activity and, at the same time, androgenic and antiandrogenic activity. This was an early formulation of the idea that we are exposed to very low levels of compounds that are likely to have a variety of endocrine actions, some reinforcing one another and others working in opposite directions.

Other early critics dismissed the evidence from animal studies, which involved much higher levels of exposure than humans would encounter under normal conditions.[21] In assessing whether the endocrine disruption hypothesis was strong enough to include in an ambitious study of the effects of early life exposures being planned by several government agencies, Matthew Longnecker of National Institute of Environmental Health Sciences concluded that "overall the evidence supporting endocrine disruption in humans is not sufficiently strong that endocrine disruption studies should be a primary motivating factor in the NCS [National Children's Study]."[22]

\* \* \*

In the early 1990s the increasing prominence of the idea that estrogenic substances in the environment might be having important effects on health coincided with intense concern and activism regarding breast cancer. Decades of research on breast cancer indicated that the main factors influencing a woman's risk—for the majority of women who lack a family history of the disease—were her age and her reproductive history. However, breast cancer advocates pointed to the increasing incidence rates of the disease in preceding decades and lobbied for research into chemical exposures that might have played a role. One of the initial targets of research was the organochlorine pesticide dichlorodiphenyltrichloroethane, or DDT, which had been widely used following World War II but which was banned for agricultural use in the United States in 1972. The most common type of breast cancer is fueled by the body's own estrogen, and it was reasoned that exposure to estrogenic compounds in the environment could also stimulate breast cancer. Interest in DDT was justified on the basis that it accumulates in fat tissue, bears a structural resemblance to DES, and exerts hormonal effects.[23] Furthermore, the International Agency for Research on Cancer had classified DDT as a "possible human carcinogen." Tests in animals indicated, however, that DDT and its analogs are much weaker estrogens compared to the body's natural estrogen—between one thousand- and one million-fold weaker.[24] It was also known that since DDT was banned for most uses in 1972, levels of the compound had decreased markedly in food and in human tissues.

So it is important to realize that the evidence in favor of DDT as a compound that might be contributing to breast cancer was relatively weak. However, a number of small epidemiologic studies had been published by the early 1990s spurring interest in this question. Then, in 1993, an article appeared in the prestigious *Journal of the National Cancer Institute* that had an enormous impact.

The study made use of stored blood samples from New York University's Women's Health Study, a prospective study designed to investigate the role of diet and hormones in the development of cancer, to measure DDT, its main metabolite dichlorodiphenyldichloroethylene (DDE), and PCBs in women diagnosed with breast cancer and women free of the disease.[25] The analysis showed that, after controlling for potential confounding factors, women with the highest blood level of DDE were nearly four times more likely to have developed breast cancer compared to women with the lowest blood level. No association was found with PCB levels. In their discussion the authors referred to the "strong association" of DDE with breast cancer risk and cautioned that, "given the widespread dissemination of organochlorines in the environment, these findings have immediate and far-reaching implications for public health intervention worldwide." An editorial accompanying the paper referred to it as a "wake-up call for further urgent research,"[26] and the National Cancer Institute and the National Institute of Environmental Health Sciences set up special programs to encourage research on DDT and other organochlorine compounds and breast cancer.

From the vantage point of twenty years, it is easier to see the *JNCI* paper in perspective, but at the time it was seized on by some as providing tangible evidence that an environmental exposure might indeed play a role in breast cancer. In reality, the paper had a number of weaknesses that should have tempered the response to it.[27] These included the small number of women who developed breast cancer (only fifty-eight cases); the fact that these cancers were diagnosed shortly after enrollment (and therefore some women may already have had breast cancer when the study began); and, finally, the fact that the dose-response relationship between DDE level and breast cancer was somewhat ambiguous and unstable due to the small numbers involved. All this should have led to a more guarded assessment of the paper.

Spurred by the *JNCI* paper, under the auspices of the National Cancer Institute and the National Institute of Environmental Health Sciences, new studies were initiated, and existing datasets were analyzed. As a result, over the following decade, several dozen analyses of the DDT/DDE and breast cancer association were published. These new studies—many of them larger and more rigorous—carried out in different populations showed no hint of an association of DDT exposure and risk of breast cancer. In 2004 a meta-analysis of the studies was published showing that the initial result—the fourfold increase in risk—appeared to be an anomaly and was not borne out by the subsequent studies.[28] In fact, when the studies were compiled and analyzed together, there was no evidence of an increased risk due to increased blood levels of DDT.[29]

The point is that the DDT–breast cancer hypothesis was never strongly supported. It was pursued because DDT/DDE could be measured in blood and because blood levels were believed to indicate something about long-term exposure in the past. The early results got a lot of attention and reinforced the belief of advocates and some members of the scientific/regulatory community that the environment must be playing a role in breast cancer. In retrospect, however, the DDT–breast cancer story can be seen as an instance of looking under the lamppost for one's keys, not because one dropped them there but because that is where the light is. At the same time, the search for effects of endocrine disrupting chemicals was to broaden out to encompass a wide range of other chemicals and potential biological effects.

While many studies focused on exposures measured in midlife in relation to breast cancer risk, at the same time a reassessment was taking place regarding environmental exposures and their contribution to breast cancer and other diseases. Several observations served as touchstones for this reassessment. First was the well-established fact that an earlier age at menarche was associated with an increased risk of breast cancer. This is usually explained by the fact that the earlier the onset of menarche and the later the onset of menopause, the longer a woman's breasts are exposed to the proliferative effects of ovarian hormones (principally estrogen). A striking demographic trend is the decline in the average age at menarche in the United States over the past 150 years from 17 to about 12 years, a trend that has accompanied improvements in living standards and nutrition. This trend and the trend toward having fewer children are themselves correlated with increasing breast cancer rates. A second observation was that, among women exposed to radiation from the atomic bomb dropped on Hiroshima, the greatest increase in breast cancer was seen in those who had been in their teens, whereas those who were adults had a much more modest increase in risk. A third, seminal, finding was the ability of DES therapy given to pregnant women to cause cancer in their daughters when they reached maturity. These observations were part of a growing recognition of the possibility that diseases occurring in adulthood may have important roots in early life. They pointedly suggested that environmental exposures may have their greatest impact during critical periods of development, including the prenatal period and puberty.[30] These insights have led to a new generation of studies following cohorts of girls through menarche to examine both lifestyle and environmental exposures in relation to breast development as well as experimental studies in animal models to understand how the timing of exposure to specific chemicals influences the mammary gland and the development of mammary tumors. Much of this work is being conducted under the auspices of the National Institute of Environmental Health Sciences.[31]

Since no studies have followed girls from birth or prepuberty for decades to see who developed breast cancer—an undertaking that would require unimaginable resources—it remains very much an open question whether exposures in utero, during puberty, or in adolescence—and, if so, which ones—influence a woman's risk of breast cancer.

In the present state of knowledge a major source of information concerning the health effects of synthetic estrogens comes from the DES experience. Although this experience is routinely cited by researchers interested in the health effects of chemicals in the environment, its real significance is rarely brought out. DES is a highly potent synthetic estrogen that is structurally similar to, and as strong as, the natural hormone estradiol. DES was administered to pregnant women as a drug to prevent miscarriage in the middle decades of the twentieth century in doses in the micrograms per kilogram of body weight per day range. These doses were escalated during the course of the pregnancy. DES was subsequently shown to cause breast cancer in exposed women as well as congenital malformations of the reproductive tract in their male and female offspring exposed in utero, including adenocarcinoma of the vagina in daughters. This contrasts with exposures to environmental contaminants measured in nanograms per kilogram of body weight—that is, to trace-level exposures that are far weaker in binding to the estrogen receptor. When the difference between these two very different exposure situations is ignored or suppressed, a critical opportunity for understanding is lost.

\* \* \*

Because breast cancer is a disease that, for the most part, occurs in older women, the attempt to link early exposures to the development of the disease is extremely challenging. In contrast, a number of male reproductive disorders occur earlier in life. These include the relatively common birth defects known as "cryptorchidism" and "hypospadias." The former refers to a condition in which one or both testes have not descended (i.e., remain within the body cavity); the latter refers to the displaced opening of the urethra along the shaft of the penis rather than at the tip. In addition to these conditions, testicular cancer tends to occur in young male adults. Finally, as noted in the opening of this chapter, variations in sperm number and quality had prompted questions about a possible decline in male fertility. The four anomalies of the male reproductive system were sometimes grouped under the label "testicular dysgenesis syndrome," or TDS.

If, in fact, sperm numbers and quality were undergoing a drastic decline worldwide, this might provide hard evidence that some exposure that had accompanied modern life—and possibly exposure to estrogenic compounds in the environment—was the culprit. Responding to the *BMJ* meta-analysis of 1992 showing declining sperm counts and, more generally, to the endocrine disruption hypothesis, researchers attempted to clarify trends in male reproductive anomalies and identify their causative factors. Over the past fifteen years, as more data have become available, the picture has changed dramatically.[32] It turned out that the participation rate in studies of semen quality, relied on in the Copenhagen paper, was quite low ("30% is regarded as good"[33]), casting doubt on the representativeness of the findings from these studies. When trends in sperm count were analyzed in studies from centers with higher-quality data, it was found that there was substantial variation in different places and differences in the trend over time. For example, data from Paris indicated that semen quality had deteriorated between 1973 and 1992, and similar evidence came from Ghent and Edinburgh. However, no evidence of a decline was found in data from Toulouse, France, or Finland, or five areas in the United States. Thus, rather than supporting the pattern of a universal decline worldwide from some common baseline, later studies indicated that there was wide variation from place to place, even within the same country.

A fundamental problem with the *BMJ* meta-analysis was that the researchers had compared data obtained from one country at one time with data from other countries obtained at other points in time.[34] The data for the early years were heavily weighted by data from New York City, whereas later studies were largely from less developed countries and from Europe.[35] In other words, the researchers were not comparing like with like. Commenting on the paper, Larry Lipshultz, a professor of urology at the Baylor College of Medicine in Houston, said that the comparison performed in the meta-analysis "would be okay if there were no such thing as geographic variation in sperm counts."[36] In the words of Michael Joffe, a specialist in human fertility at Imperial College London, "The idea of a simultaneous decline, with similar levels across wide swaths of the globe, needs to be abandoned."[37]

But the problem with examining trends in sperm number and quality goes much deeper. As Harry Fisch of Columbia University pointed out in a penetrating analysis of the issue, sperm number, semen volume, and sperm morphology vary not only by geographic region and between individuals but also within individuals.[38] Sperm count and quality are influenced by the following factors: time since last ejaculation, scrotal temperature, prolonged sitting, season, smoking, and drug use. These factors were not controlled for and received little attention in discussions of declining sperm count.

Fisch went on to emphasize the biased sampling in the studies included in the *BMJ* meta-analysis and itemized six "major weaknesses." One of these is the comparison of data from different countries at different times, as mentioned above. Fisch demonstrated that when the data from Carlsen and colleagues were reanalyzed accounting for geographic variation, no decline in sperm counts was seen. Furthermore, according to Fisch, thirty-one studies that were published following the Carlsen study attempted to address important methodological problems. Of these newer studies, six showed clear evidence of a decline in sperm counts; sixteen studies (including ten times as many subjects as in the studies showing evidence of a decline) showed either no change or an increase; and the remaining studies showed ambiguous results.

Fisch commented that, "far from being a worldwide and well-proved phenomenon, declines in semen quality are, at best, a highly local phenomenon with an unknown cause and, at worst, a collective artifact arising from the observation of a highly variable physical attribute (sperm counts) with a relatively low-resolution tool (retrospective analysis of non-randomized study populations)." In view of its many flaws, he argued that the *BMJ* meta-analysis "warrants its exclusion from any review of data supporting a decline." [39]

Attempts to demonstrate links between other aspects of male reproductive capacity and exposure to endocrine disrupting chemicals proved similarly problematic.

Whatever the vagaries of sperm concentration and quality and the many factors (climate, lifestyle, exposure to infectious organisms, environmental exposures, genetics, in addition to those mentioned by Fisch) that may influence them, sperm number and quality are only weakly associated with male fertility.[40] Therefore any impact of a decline in sperm quality on male fertility is likely to be small. Like trends in sperm concentration, trends in fertility also show variation by place. Studies in Europe and the United States actually indicated an overall rising trend in fertility, casting added doubt on the significance of the sperm count data.[41] Rather than drawing any conclusions, Joffe concluded his discussion by emphasizing the urgent need for research that sheds light on behavioral factors that influence fertility.

Regarding testicular cancer, Joffe has argued that the epidemiology of the disease is not consistent with exposure to chemicals in the environment beginning in the post–World War II period. Reliable statistics are available regarding testicular cancer in developed countries. This cancer typically occurs in young men, between the ages of 20 and 45. Its incidence has increased dramatically (between three- and fourfold) in European and certain other populations. In England and Wales, the rise in incidence started in 1920, and in northern Europe around midcentury. Since there is clear evidence that testicular cancer is initiated early in life and possibly in utero, this suggests strongly that early life events at the beginning of the twentieth century or the late nineteenth century are germane to the rise in incidence. This makes the hypothesis that exposure to chemicals in the post–World War II environment rather unconvincing. Joffe concluded that "clearly the factors(s) responsible for the rise in testicular cancer in the 20th century do(es) not explain all of the observed variation in male reproductive system impairment."[42]

Unlike the situation regarding testicular cancer, reliable data on trends in hypospadias and cryptorchidism are scarce, making inferences about their causes difficult. A review of data from twenty-nine registries that monitor a total of four million births per year around the world revealed wide intercountry variation in rates of these conditions.[43] There was a suggestion of an increase in hypospadias in more affluent countries, which appeared to end in the mid-1980s. The author pointed out that a number of artifacts might account for the apparent increase, including changes in the definition of hypospadias and changes in physician registration practices. There was no indication of an increase in cryptorchidism since 1970. Thus, in spite of common claims that the rates of these conditions are increasing, more systematic examinations do not support this impression. Furthermore, there is no clear evidence that low-level environmental exposures contribute to these conditions.[44]

Joffe concluded his assessment with the words, "In summary, a thorough review of the evidence leads to the conclusion that the endocrine disruption hypothesis cannot explain the main features of the rise in testicular cancer or more broadly of TDS [testicular dysgenesis syndrome]."[45] As we shall see, others who have tried to take a broad view, putting the diverse research findings in perspective, have reached similar conclusions.

\* \* \*

After more than two decades of research and thousands of scientific papers devoted to endocrine disruption, the field has become embroiled in a bewildering scientific and political controversy focused on an unlikely culprit—a compound that has been in wide use for over fifty years. Bisphenol A, or BPA, is a carbon-based compound first synthesized by a Russian chemist in 1891. Since the late 1950s it has been widely used in the manufacture of polycarbonate plastic bottles and in the epoxy resins used to line food and beverage containers. The latter use has proved highly effective in preventing illness due to food spoilage. In recent years BPA has found its way into a wide variety of products, including medical equipment, bike helmets, reading glasses, CDs, bullet-proof glass, smart phones, flat-screen televisions, and thermal sales receipt paper.

In the early 1930s the British biochemist Edward Charles Dodds had observed that, owing to its resemblance to the natural estrogen estradiol, BPA had the ability to mimic estrogen, triggering estrogen pathways within the body; however, he determined that BPA was thirty-seven thousand times weaker than estradiol.[46] But it was not until the 1990s that the first scientific papers investigating possible health effects of BPA exposure started appearing, and the chemical became a major focus of scientific research only in the late 1990s. Another ten years elapsed before BPA seized the attention of the public owing to reports that it could leach out of plastic bottles, food containers, and "sippy cups" used by infants, leading to calls for regulating and banning BPA in consumer products.[47]

One paper in particular had sparked scientific interest in BPA as a chemical that could disrupt normal development. In 1997 Susan C. Nagel and colleagues at the University of Missouri reported that exposing fetal mice to a low dose of BPA resulted in estrogenic activity.[48] Specifically, prostate weight was increased in male mice at six months of age following exposure of the pregnant dams to BPA during gestation. The paper was from the laboratory of Frederick vom Saal, a biologist who had done important work on fetal exposure to hormones and who was to become a leading figure asserting the dangers of BPA to human health. The Nagel paper was to stimulate a cascade of papers from vom Saal and other groups, which appeared to show evidence of a wide variety of adverse effects from exposure to low doses of BPA that had been assumed to be safe. From the 1960s until the late 1990s only a handful of scientific papers had appeared each year on the health effects of BPA. In 1997 the number increased to 10; in 2005, there were 65 publications; and in 2013, 199.

These studies have involved many different test systems and mechanisms of hormonal action at different stages of development. In addition to experimental studies in animals and cell culture, there have been many epidemiologic studies examining associations of BPA levels (usually measured in urine) and health outcomes including diabetes, obesity, breast cancer, heart disease, and behavioral abnormalities.[49]

Since the late 1990s there has been a pointed controversy concerning the interpretation of the results of both the experimental and the epidemiological studies on BPA. As research findings have accumulated, rather than resolving key differences, the controversy has only intensified, and the opposing positions have become more entrenched. This has led to the existence of two camps with drastically divergent interpretations of the same body of evidence. For the purposes of identifying the two groups, I will refer to them as the "proponents" or "advocates" of BPA as an endocrine disruptor and "opponents" or "critics" of the hypothesis, respectively. Some of the leading figures among the proponents are Frederick vom Saal and his group at the University of Missouri; Ana Soto, Carlos Sonnenschein, and Laura Vandenberg of Tufts University; Thomas Zoeller of the University of Massachusetts at Amherst; Niels Skakkebaek of Copenhagen's Royal Hospital; and Linda Birnbaum, the director of the National Institute of Environmental Health Sciences. Scientists in the opposition include Stephen Safe of Texas A&M University, Daniel Doerge of the FDA's National Center for Toxicological Research, Justin Teeguarden of Pacific Northwest National Laboratory, Rochelle Tyl of Research Triangle Institute, and Richard Sharpe of the University of Edinburgh.

The two camps differ on technical issues, the overall interpretation of the available evidence, the most fundamental principles of toxicology, and, finally, philosophy regarding regulation and the basis for regulatory action (i.e., invocation of the precautionary principle). It would be hard to imagine a more complete disjunction between two groups examining the same body of evidence.

Key methodological issues dividing the two camps include (1) the level of BPA exposure at which effects are observed and the pattern of effects at different exposure levels and whether there is a threshold below which no effects are observed; (2) the importance of different routes of exposure (dermal and inhalation versus ingestion); (3) metabolism and excretion of BPA following exposure by different routes; (4) the relevance of animal models to the human exposure situation; and (5) the validity of measuring BPA in blood and the issue of contamination. Underlying these specific points of disagreement are the questions of whether humans are exposed to truly significant levels of BPA and whether any biological effects can be reliably attributed to this exposure.

A fundamental principle of toxicology is that "the dose makes the poison." This principle lies behind the "dose-response relationship" that is seen for most toxins, that is, the higher the dose to which humans or test animals are exposed, the higher likelihood of observing an effect. Examples of the dose-response are seen in the effects of smoking cigarettes (the greater the number of cigarettes smoked per day, the greater the risk of lung cancer and other diseases caused by smoking), exposure to ionizing radiation, and exposure to lead. The assumption of a dose-response underlies environmental regulation. Advocates of endocrine disruption argue that this model does not apply to the action of hormones, and they posit the existence of what they call a "nonmonotonic dose-response" model or "U-shaped dose-response," meaning that effects can occur at low levels of exposure, whereas there may be no observable effect or a weaker effect at an intermediate or higher level of exposure. The advocates argue that there are plausible mechanisms that can explain this unorthodox dose-response.[50] If this contention were correct, it would require a major rethinking of toxicology.[51]

Regarding the significance of BPA concentrations measured in human populations, the advocates argue that the levels of the compound measured in urine and in blood in certain studies represent significant exposure, and that these levels correspond to exposure levels at which detrimental effects are observed in experimental animal studies.

Although it is generally agreed that greater than 90 percent of BPA exposure comes from ingesting food that has absorbed the chemical from packaging, the advocates argue that other "routes of exposure" may be important, including inhalation of air or dust containing BPA, dermal absorption of BPA from thermal paper receipts, and bathing in contaminated water. Furthermore, they argue that these alternative routes of exposure are likely to result in significant levels of the active compound since they bypass the liver, where most BPA is deactivated. This would mean that the burden of BPA in the body has been underestimated owing to the focus on ingestion as the main route of exposure. Advocates also emphasize that BPA in the mother's circulation is transferred to the developing fetus through the placenta, thereby potentially posing a serious danger.

In their position papers, advocates of endocrine disruption make what appear to be plausible and cogent arguments. However, reading through their papers claiming significant adverse effects of BPA exposure, one is struck by a number of features of their style of argumentation. First, there is little concern for, or attention to, overall quality or methodology of the different studies for its own sake. Rather, methodology seems to become an issue only when the proponents are defending the results of studies that are in line with their hypothesis. Thus little or no attention is paid to experimental design, adequate sample size, appropriateness of the experimental system to real-world exposure, or replication of results.

Second, not surprisingly, there is a tendency to cite work by the authors themselves and like-minded scientists from other groups. It is striking, however, that there is virtually no acknowledgment of any results that go counter to their hypothesis. It is highly unusual in science that all findings line up perfectly in support of one's hypothesis, and it is essential to attempt to understand the reasons for apparent contradictions, in order to make progress.

Third, there is a narrowness of focus, by which I mean that virtually no recognition is given to the fact that in comparison to low-level exposures to environmental contaminants, there are other exposures that are likely to greatly outweigh them, namely, obesity, the body's natural hormones, and phytoestrogens in the diet, which are many orders of magnitude more potent than what is being investigated. These factors, as well as others, such as maternal smoking and use of certain medications, would be likely to dwarf the effects of what is being studied. However, there is no attempt to put exposure to endocrine disruptors in a broader context.

Fourth, the proponents' publications tend to refer to the increasing frequency of various diseases or conditions and imply that endocrine disruption is playing a role. In fact, as we have seen, in spite of decades of research there is no firm evidence to support a role of endocrine disrupting chemicals in these diseases.

Essentially, it appears that the proponents are expressing their *belief* in the endocrine disruption hypothesis very much in the vein of the Wingspread statement of 1991. But all they have to point to are questionable results that have not been replicated, and they studiously avoid acknowledging that there is no firm or consistent evidence of an effect. Finally, there is a tendency to favor certain types of research (particularly academic research funded by the National Institute of Environmental Health Sciences) and to impugn the motives of those whose results they disagree with, implying that research funded by industry or government agencies such as the EPA and the FDA is automatically flawed.[52] Once one becomes aware of these stylistic features, one begins to suspect that the proponents of endocrine disruption have a predetermined goal, and that, rather than judging studies on their merits and taking only the best evidence into account, they are wedded to results that support their position.

If one's investment in a hypothesis is so powerful that one loses the ability to assess studies dispassionately and objectively—independent of whether the results conform to one's hypothesis—it is easy to be misled. There are many points at which bias can creep into the design of an experiment or its interpretation. For example, the earliest experiment to raise the question of "low-dose" effects of BPA by Nagel and vom Saal in 1997 involved giving BPA in drinking water to pregnant mice during the prenatal and immediately postnatal periods. To examine effects on prostate weight in male offspring, they randomly selected one adult male from each of seven litters.

Studies attempting to replicate these findings have shown that there is substantial variability in prostate weight within a single litter. In one such study, when all members of the litter were included in the analysis, no association was found between BPA exposure and prostate weight.[53] In fact, the study by Nagel and colleagues has never been successfully repeated; however, this does not deter the advocates from citing it as important evidence of endocrine disruption. This is just one example that drives home a point that is fundamental to research studies but virtually never gets attention when results are presented to the public. That is, what data were collected and how they were collected can determine the result obtained. We saw something similar in the claims of a drastic decline in sperm counts, which was most likely due to a biased selection of data included in the meta-analysis published in *BMJ* in 1992. Many similar pitfalls affecting studies of endocrine disruption have been pointed out in the literature.[54]

As basic research studies focused on particular test systems and mechanisms and studies attempting to assess BPA exposure and its effects in human populations have piled up, some very high-quality studies have appeared, raising damaging questions about BPA as a "model endocrine disruptor." These well-designed studies provide data on BPA exposure, metabolism, and excretion in rats and monkeys in utero and postnatally, and on heavy BPA exposure in humans. And they indicate that consumer products contain little BPA, and leaching from the container or packaging into the food is minimal.[55] Moreover, although most U.S. residents are exposed, actual exposures are very low—more than 99 percent of ingested BPA is efficiently metabolized and excreted. And this is true even in newborns.[56] Crucially, these studies measured both free and bound BPA—only the free compound can have biological effects.

In a real-world experiment to determine the impact of heavy BPA exposure on blood and urine levels, Justin Teeguarden of Pacific Northwest National Laboratory and colleagues had twenty volunteers eat meals rich in canned foods and analyzed BPA in blood and urine samples collected over a twenty-four-hour period.[57] The experimental diet was designed to put the subjects in the ninety-fifth percentile for BPA exposure in the United States. In spite of their high exposure, free BPA was not detectable in any of 320 blood samples using a highly sensitive method, indicating that the compound was rapidly absorbed and rapidly excreted. This confirmed how low actual human exposures are, even under high-dose conditions.

To make sense of the contradictory findings and conflicting interpretations bedeviling the field, Teeguarden and colleagues carried out a reevaluation of published studies that had reported serum BPA concentrations to determine whether they could plausibly be causing estrogen-mediated effects.[58] Their analysis included data from ninety-three published studies of more than thirty thousand individuals in nineteen countries across all life stages. The authors used four different methods to calculate serum BPA concentrations. These methods took into account what is known about the correlation between urinary and blood BPA levels, different routes of exposure, and levels predicted by a validated human pharmacokinetic model (that modeled how BPA is metabolized and excreted). The different methods gave a remarkably consistent picture of the range of active and inactive BPA serum levels. In the authors' words, "Typical serum BPA concentrations are orders of magnitude lower than levels measurable by modern analytical methods and below concentrations required to occupy more than 0.0009%" of major estrogen binding sites. They concluded: "Our results show limited or no potential for estrogenicity in human, and question reports of measurable BPA in human serum."

Given this impressive consistency, how was one to explain reports in the literature of blood BPA concentrations three orders of magnitude higher than those they had obtained? After ruling out a number of possible explanations, Teeguarden and colleagues concluded that the high serum BPA concentrations reported in some studies could plausibly be explained by their having been conducted in a hospital or clinic setting, where contamination of the blood samples by BPA in medical devices, including intravenous lines, could have resulted in higher BPA concentrations than what is consistently measured in the general population.[59]

This is the kind of analysis that examines all available data in order to identify the reasons behind the conflicting results cited by different groups. If the analysis by Teeguarden and colleagues is correct, this would indicate that the study results that the endocrine disruption proponents take as the cornerstone of their case (that human exposures to BPA and their effects are being missed) are actually *outliers*, that is, results that are anomalous, probably due to poor methodology, and therefore of questionable relevance to public health.

The proponents have come back stronger than ever, however, attacking the results and the arguments of their opponents and defending their own studies against all criticisms.[60] They claim that circulating levels of unconjugated BPA are higher than what is predicted by models that assume that the only relevant route of exposure is oral. They flatly reject the criticism that the high levels of BPA in blood in their favored studies are due to sample contamination. And they stress that effects of BPA exposure on the fetus and in early life have been demonstrated and are explained by the much less developed capacity of the fetus and the developing animal to metabolize the chemical.

Finally, we should note that the advocates' position is at odds with the conclusions of many national health agencies, including the U.S. FDA, the EPA, Health Canada, the European Food Safety Authority, Food Standards Australia New Zealand, and the German Federal Institute for Risk Assessment, which, after thoroughgoing assessments of the evidence, have found BPA to be safe at levels to which the general population is exposed.

* * *

In the summer of 2013 the long-standing scientific debate over endocrine disruption erupted in a new forum when a European Commission (EC) proposal to regulate endocrine disruptors was leaked. The commission's framework for its proposed regulation was based on a document drawn up under the auspices of the United Nations Development Program and the World Health Organization entitled *Endocrine Disrupting Chemicals 2012: The State of the Science*.[61] Citing the report, the European Commission document called for "appropriate policy action on the basis of the precautionary principle" to regulate endocrine disruptors as a distinct category of chemicals, even though they are already covered by existing laws concerning toxic substances. News of the EC proposal provoked an immediate and scathing response in the form of an open letter to the commission's chief scientific adviser, Anne Glover, by Daniel Dietrich of the University of Konstanz in Germany and signed by eighteen toxicology journal editors. The letter, which was published as an editorial in fourteen toxicology journals, charged the commission with planning to regulate "so-called endocrine disrupting chemicals" within a framework that was "based on virtually complete ignorance of all well-established and taught principles of pharmacology and toxicology."[62] The authors questioned why "endocrine disrupting chemicals" should be treated as a distinct category and judged by different standards from those routinely applied to any chemical. They stressed the need to take into account real-world exposure and to accept the principle of a threshold below which adverse effects are not observed. They criticized the EC framework for failing to distinguish between transient perturbations and truly adverse effects and stressed the need to base its judgments on data from human studies and whole animal experiments, rather than on data from artificial test systems (in vitro tests). The editorial further charged that the EC framework inexplicably ignored the conclusions of its own expert authority, the European Food Safety Authority, as well as those of other bodies and societies that had determined that BPA was not a hazard at levels to which people are normally exposed. Finally, they stressed the harm to science and society that will be caused by allowing the complex process of evaluating the science to be influenced by political pressures. In the following months nearly one hundred scientists signed the Dietrich editorial.

Proponents of endocrine disruption responded with a defense of the EC framework, which was also published in multiple journals. They rejected each of Dietrich and colleagues' criticisms and accused them of ignoring evidence that disruption of the endocrine system during development can lead to irreversible effects.[63] The endocrinologist Andrea Gore charged that the Dietrich editorial "seeks to foment doubt on the relevance of EDCs" and reflected "unrelenting pressure from individuals and corporations with stakes in the status quo to keep doubt alive." She characterized the events over the summer and early fall as "one of the most remarkable experiences in my career." While acknowledging that it was vital that the two communities work together on this issue, she admitted that, "It's hard to imagine these two groups sitting down and having a pleasant conversation."[64]

Owing to the unfortunate experience of pregnant women who were given the synthetic estrogen DES in the middle of the last century, we know something about the long-term effects of this compound at high doses. It took decades of following these women and their children to document the health effects from that exposure. Let's take a moment to make an obvious comparison, which, tellingly, is virtually never made by proponents of endocrine disruption. The average exposure of Americans to BPA is about 0.02 micrograms per kilogram of body weight.[65] DES, on the other hand, was given to pregnant women at doses as high as 2,000 micrograms per kilogram of body weight[66]—a difference of about five orders of magnitude. But, in addition, BPA has approximately ten-thousand-fold lower estrogenic potency compared to DES. So if we take into account both dose and potency, we are talking about a difference of nine orders of magnitude!

At the heart of this heated debate are not only starkly divergent readings of the evidence, as we have seen, but also two very different philosophies. Invocation of the precautionary principle by proponents of the endocrine disruption hypothesis sounds eminently reasonable. It simply argues that if the potential harmful effects of an action or an exposure are not fully known, one should act in such a way as to minimize any possible adverse effects. The problem is that, when applied to the question of endocrine disruption, this seemingly reasonable approach ignores the extensive scientific evidence that has accumulated over the past two decades. And, as we have seen, in order to support their contention of a hazard, proponents are forced to ignore the high-quality studies and defend results that have never been successfully replicated. An important shortcoming of the proponents' position is that it fails to distinguish between transient effects (due to the body's compensatory response to endocrine perturbations) and irreversible effects.[67] Ignoring such crucial distinctions, the proponents rely on "hazard identification," placing emphasis on the toxicity of synthetic chemicals, while ignoring "weight-of-the-evidence" assessments that take into account actual exposure in real-world situations and what is known from experiments in whole animals. Rather than "hazard identification," which ignores some of the most crucial information available (i.e., human exposure data), the critics argue that what is needed is a "risk assessment" approach that takes into account all relevant scientific information available.[68]

Doing justice to the complexity of the science on endocrine disruption and the difficulty of establishing clear-cut effects is in itself a daunting task. However, once a scientific question gets catapulted into the public arena, the science and its interpretation no longer occupy a protected realm, where the standards of scientific discourse are supposed to hold sway. Rather, the science becomes hopelessly overlaid with personal, political, and ideological associations. The French sociologist of science Bruno Latour has referred to these composite objects as *hybrids*. These overtones and associations can become as important as the science, and many will react to the narrative of the science they find most convincing and congenial based on these overtones and associations.

\* \* \*

It is important to realize that this intense controversy, which pits two camps with dramatically divergent interpretations of the same body of evidence, can exist because of the low levels of exposure; the complexity of biology, with the possibility of different effects at different stages of development; the large number of factors and exposures that can distort normal development; the differences between animal models and humans, making extrapolation from the former to the latter perilous; and the difficulty of establishing causal associations between a low-level exposure and health effects in humans. Given the depth and intensity of the controversy, its political overtones, and its far-reaching policy implications, it is difficult to see how the current impasse will get resolved any time soon.

Rather than looking for an imminent resolution of the controversy, it is more rewarding to step back from the narrow focus on "endocrine disruption" and take a wider view of the issue. It comes as a breath of fresh air when one moves from individual studies and the literature of debate to attempts to reflect critically on the experience of the past two to three decades and ask what has been learned. A number of academic researchers have been prompted by the endocrine disruption experience to write overviews that attempt to put the issue in perspective. These commentaries may bring us as close to the truth of the matter as we can get at present. Their authors do not rule out the possibility that major discoveries will be made in the future, but, for the most part, they are confident enough about the high-quality work that has been done that they are able to say that, for now, maybe enough attention has been devoted to BPA and to endocrine disruption in general and maybe it is time to look at new hypotheses. The impulse behind these overviews is to learn from the experience of the past twenty years in order to turn the page.

The critical reflections of these scientists on the endocrine disruption saga help make sense of the almost impenetrable confusion surrounding the issue. They explain how science can get hijacked and diverted by non-scientific agendas and how an issue like BPA can take on a life of its own, siphoning off enormous amounts of scarce research funds and regulatory attention.[69] By critically examining the claims and the findings regarding endocrine disruption and placing them in a broader context, these overviews take stock of what has been learned and raise the question of where one should look in the future for more productive hypotheses regarding exposures that affect human health and development. In addition to published reflections by figures involved in research on endocrine disruption, I also refer below to interviews that I conducted with a number of these figures.

Allen Wilcox, who is a senior scientist at the National Institute of Environmental Health Sciences (NIEHS), has a valuable perspective on the endocrine disruption hypothesis. His career has been devoted to the study of environmental exposures on human reproduction. In the early 1990s, motivated by the finding that DES was a transplacental carcinogen, Wilcox and colleagues formulated a number of other hypotheses about effects of DES on human health based on findings in animals and basic science.[70] He and his colleagues had what they considered the perfect research design to test these hypotheses, namely, follow-up of the randomized DES clinical trial done at the University of Chicago in the early 1950s. (Wilcox commented to me that "random allocation of the exposure of interest is a luxury few epi-demiologists ever get.") None of their hypotheses was borne out by the data, "and we published six (!) negative papers." He acknowledged that there are of course many differences between DES and environmental estrogens, and "there may be important ED [endocrine disruption] effects yet to be dis-covered—but I have to admit that my own negative studies made me a bit skeptical about ED effects reported in less rigorous studies."[71]

Earlier I cited Michael Joffe's views on the possibility that exposure to low-level estrogenic chemicals in the environment could be playing a role in male reproductive abnormalities. At the end of one of his critical reviews, Joffe commented on the impact of attention to the endocrine dis-ruption hypothesis on the ability to conduct original science in his area:

> One hypothesis to explain the deterioration in the aspects of male reproductive health grouped together as TDS [testicular dysgenesis syndrome] is that it is due to some form of endocrine disruption or modulation. This has been highly influential since the early 1990s, to the extent that it has not only driven out discussion of other hypoth-eses, but has also dominated the debate about the male reproductive system—major research programs on endocrine disruption were ini-tiated in the USA and Europe, and in most countries it was only pos-sible to carry out research on the epidemiology of male reproduction if the project could be presented as a test of the endocrine disruption hypothesis.[72]

Richard Sharpe, who specializes in male reproductive function, occu-pies an unusual position in the endocrine disruption controversy. Since the early 1990s he has taken seriously the possibility that significant exposure to chemicals in the environment could play a role in human disease, but at the same time he has been uncompromising as a scientist and has been a severe critic of the poor quality of much on the work on endocrine dis-ruption. In a sense he has taken both sides in the controversy. For these reasons, his perspective on the science and on the factors that led to the inflation of the issue is especially worth hearing. In an e-mail he wrote:

> In my opinion the big problem in this area is that it has become an "industry," sucking in huge amounts of funding in ways that have become self-serving and self-supporting. So many people's labs, ca-reers and funding are dependent on the "threat" from EDCs being real and important, that they do not look in any other direction for

explanations. In science that is a danger that I always teach students/ young scientists about, because it can cost you your career if it turns out you are wrong (and most of the time we are). To borrow a term used all too often by the EDC researchers, there is a huge influence of "vested interest," not from industry in this case (although that is omnipresent), but from the EDC research community.[73]

Based on his own experience, he can see how the pressures on scientists (publications, publicity, getting grants, career advancement) can distort the path they take. He wrote that "in retrospect I consider that circumstances helped me because I ended up disproving my own hypothesis/ideas (on the potential impact of environmental oestrogens on male reproductive disorders) early on in the ED saga." And he went on to make a crucial distinction: "plus I was lucky that the question that drove me was 'what causes these disorders?' not 'how do EDCs cause these disorders?' Such a simple difference, but it takes your thought processes in a very different direction."[74]

Perhaps the strongest and most penetrating comments on the mechanisms that allowed anomalous research results on BPA to obscure more rigorous research findings come from Daniel Doerge of the Food and Drug Administration's National Center for Toxicological Research. In response to a question from me, Doerge wrote:

As long as investigators see that others can successfully use a strategy that is fundamentally uncritical (i.e., by only pursuing evidence of toxicity and disregarding evidence against their chosen hypothesis, disregarding human exposure, inadequate experimental design), why shouldn't they pile on the bandwagon? I think the BPA episode is instructive in how a well-disciplined, but unprincipled, group of academic investigators spun a distorted version of reality. In this alternate reality, the tools of science are given over to the political realm, where distorted concepts and inflammatory rhetoric become weapons to destroy individuals espousing opposing conclusions. When such a self-interested group gains access to the levers of a large national funding agency, the chaos can continue for an extended time. This model is obviously applicable to any other chemical entity that a fearful pubic can be driven to focus on.[75]

If BPA has been a costly distraction/diversion that has consumed hundreds of millions of research dollars and massive regulatory attention and generated widespread public concern and confusion, what targets should researchers interested in environmental contributions (in the broadest possible sense) to disease focus on?

Doerge emphasized that, unlike BPA, which is a very weak estrogen and is rapidly metabolized, more persistent toxins that entail long-lasting exposure and accumulation in the body are more plausible targets of research. He pointed out that there are clearly dangerous chemicals in the environment, like inorganic arsenic, that should receive more attention. In addition, he feels that TCDD (dioxin) is "problematic" because of its highly persistent nature in the body and its toxic potency in many experimental animals. Doerge has devoted much of his career to the toxicity and carcinogenicity of compounds in the diet (this is what motivated him to turn his attention to BPA, whose principal source is the diet). He thinks that acrylamide—a compound that is formed when starchy foods such as potato chips and French fries are heated higher than 248° Fahrenheit—is "interesting" since animal studies provide strong evidence of carcinogenicity. And he thinks that it is probably a human carcinogen. He notes, however, that because exposure to acrylamide is so widespread and is essentially unavoidable in the general population (factors that also make it difficult to study epidemiologically), there is probably little that can be done to reduce the risk at the population level.[76]

When I asked Richard Sharpe what he thought are more worthwhile research questions in the field of reproductive disorders, he said he would answer in a "roundabout way." He told me about John Sumpter, a professor of aquatic ecotoxicology in Britain, who did seminal work on estrogens in sewage effluent and the induction of intersex in fish. Sumpter, Sharpe told me, gives a superb talk in which he tells of his research starting in the early 1990s devoted to alkylphenols, which had been identified as being weakly estrogenic and which were clearly released into river water. It was only after ten years of work and large amounts of money that he and his colleagues finally "nail[ed] the culprit, and of course it turned out to be ethinyl estradiol/other potent synthetic estrogens" (i.e., from oral contraceptives). Sharpe said that Sumpter would end his talk by saying that in light of this discovery, "You would think that we would have indulged in some intelligent thinking, but sadly we appear not to have done so across the ED world."[77]

Sharpe continued:

With this example in mind, I often in talks pose the question, "if we were to start from scratch in looking for what sorts of exogenous factors might impact reproductive development via hormonal perturbations, where would be the most logical place to start looking? Should we start with very weakly active compounds that are present in the environment (i.e., in low/very low levels) and which are readily metabolized or should we start with compounds that are designed to be bioactive and resistant to metabolism/breakdown and which we are exposed to intentionally in high amounts (I'm talking about pharmaceuticals or, less likely perhaps, certain components of diet)?" As you know, the answer is that only the unlikely option has been investigated in the main, even though it is illogical.

Sharpe told me that he is now taking the logical route and for the past three years has been examining the effects of pharmaceuticals taken by pregnant women on the fetus and the developing child. This work is producing evidence of real effects including cryptorchidism and neurobehavioral effects. He doesn't claim that these effects explain all reproductive disorders, but "what it does shout out is that we have been looking in very much the wrong direction, the lack of intelligent thinking once again."

The endocrine disruption story and particularly the BPA saga are cautionary tales of what happens when science is hijacked by people who use the power and the prestige of science to scare the public, work the media, and pressure health agencies to pile on the bandwagon and fund work that stands little chance of advancing our knowledge about the complex processes involved in normal development and disease. The appeal to the public and the media—science by press release—in an area as conflicted and as contested as the endocrine disruption hypothesis short-circuits the crucial process of working out the science. We need fewer but better studies that can help elucidate the key underlying issues, and eventually we need to reach a scientific consensus on what the evidence shows. Until then, we need to be aware of both the scientific reasons for the impasse as well as all the extrascientific agendas that get imposed on the science. Certainly, as a number of people pointed out to me, some responsibility lies with the media, which is always ready to retail scary reports about a threat lurking in the recesses of our daily lives. But ultimately, as Doerge and all the scientists who insist on maintaining a critical stance stressed, this issue has to do with the conduct of science in the area of the "environment" and human health. Doerge, along with scientists at the highest reaches of the National Institutes of Health, see the need for a total overhaul of the process by which scientific research is conceived, evaluated, funded, reviewed for publication, and published. As Doerge commented to me, "When we are not the most critical of our own data we defer that obligation to others."[78]

# 6

## Deadly Remedy
### A Mysterious Disease, a Medicinal Herb, and the Recognition of a Worldwide Public Health Threat

Just because something is natural it does not mean that it is good, and just because something is unnatural it does not mean that it is bad. Arsenic, cobra poison, nuclear radiation, earthquakes, and the Ebola virus can all be found in nature, whereas vaccines, spectacles, and artificial hips are all man-made.

—SIMON SINGH AND EDZARD ERNST

As head of the nephrology service at the Erasmus Hospital of the Free University of Brussels, Dr. Jean-Louis Vanherweghem had seen many cases of chronic kidney disease. Usually this condition occurs in older people and is most commonly associated with diabetes and hypertension. But he and his colleagues were at loss when, in the early 1990s, relatively young women started showing up at hospitals in the city with unexplained and rapidly progressing kidney disease. Tests showed anemia and elevated creatinine levels, indicating that the kidneys were not doing their job of filtering toxins and waste products from the blood. In a matter of months, many of the women went on to develop life-threatening end-stage renal disease and had to go on dialysis or have a kidney transplant. Most were in their forties, and none had a history of medical conditions that would have put them at increased risk.

One day, as Dr. Vanherweghem came out of his office into the waiting room, he noticed that several of the women were chatting. Asking how they were acquainted, he learned that they had all attended the same weight-loss clinic. Over the following months and years, the number of young women with kidney damage coming in to his and other clinics in the city continued to grow.

To pinpoint the cause of this epidemic of kidney failure, Vanherwe-ghem and colleagues contacted nephrology centers throughout Brussels to identify all cases of renal failure occurring in women under fifty. In their initial report published in the *Lancet* in 1993, they described the results of nine cases of nephropathy in young women and examined details of the weight-loss regimen and the various medications the women were taking.[1] They learned that the weight-loss clinic had been in operation for fifteen years—from 1975 until May 1990—with no apparent ill effects. During that period the slimming regimen had consisted of a mixture of thirteen compounds given in capsule form or by injection. In May 1990, however, the regime had been modified, with the addition of two Chinese herbs believed to be *Stephania tetendra* and *Magnolia officinalis*. This regimen was in place for the next two years. While the authors were appropriately circumspect regarding the specific ingredient responsible for the kidney damage, they emphasized the striking connection between the unusual pathology and a slimming treatment involving Chinese herbs.

As time went on, more women from the weight-loss clinic sought medical attention for renal disease, and the syndrome was given the name "Chinese herbs nephropathy."[2] Early descriptions of the renal pathology had been based on biopsies, which provided only very small amounts of tissue. But in 1994 Jean-Pierre Cosyns, a pathologist at the hospital of the Catholic University of Louvain, across town from the Erasmus Hospital, used three whole kidneys from patients with Chinese herbs nephropathy to give the first detailed description of what the pathology looked like.[3] He described a distinctive fibrosis, or scarring, of the renal tubules, the structures that are responsible for reabsorbing electrolytes and excreting wastes. The fibrosis is most prominent in the outer layers of the kidney (the cortex) and works its way inward. Something similar is seen only with cadmium poisoning. Cosyns pointed out that, on "morphological and clinical grounds," the lesions seen in the Belgian women were "very similar to those described in Balkan endemic nephropathy," and he and his coauthors suggested that a "common agent" might be involved in both diseases.[4] In addition, both Cosyns and the nephrologists at Erasmus Hospital noted changes in the cells of the renal pelvis (the funnel-shaped part of the kidney where urine collects after filtration from the blood) and the ureters signifying the early stages of cancer. In a separate paper in 1994, he reported the first case of urothelial malignancy among women with Chinese herbs nephropathy.[5] "Urothelial" refers to the distinctive type of cells lining the urinary tract, including the renal pelvis, ureters, and bladder. This cell type is distinct from the type of cells in the renal cortex, in which 90 percent of *kidney cancer* arises.

By 1995 eighty cases of Chinese herbs nephropathy in Brussels had come to light. Because exposed women appeared to be at high risk of developing urothelial cancer as well as kidney failure, Vanherweghem recommended regular cystoscopic examinations and the prophylactic removal of the kidneys and ureters in all his patients with end-stage Chinese herbs nephropathy. By the time he and his colleagues published their findings regarding cancer in the *New England Journal of Medicine* in 2000, thirty-nine patients had agreed to undergo prophylactic surgery.[6] Microscopic examination of the upper urothelial tissues from eighteen of the patients revealed cancer, and those of another nineteen patients showed mild to moderate urothelial dysplasia, a precursor to cancer. Thus the clinicians' aggressive response proved to be well-founded.

Further investigation revealed the exact nature of the change in the mixture of powdered herbs used at the weight-loss clinic that had occurred in May 1990. Instead of *Stefania tetendra* and *Magnolia*, the company that supplied the Chinese herbs had substituted *Aristolochia*. The tragic mix-up was facilitated by the similarity of the names for the two herbs in Chinese.[7] *Aristolochia* is *fangchi*, whereas *Stephania* is *fangji*. In contrast to the benign *Stephania*, *Aristolochia fangchi* contains aristolochic acid—a powerful nephrotoxin and carcinogen—which belongs to the class of chemicals called nitrophenanthrenes. (Diesel fuel contains nitrophenantrenes.)

*Aristolochiaceae* are a family of flowering plants with over five hundred species, which are found in diverse climates worldwide. The European birthwort (*Aristolochia clematitis*) is so named because its flower resembles a birth canal. *Aristolochiaceae* have been used in different cultures in the ancient Mediterranean world, in Europe, South America, India, and China, and in other countries in East Asia going back at least two thousand years.[8] *Aristolochia clematitis* was highly valued as a medicinal plant in ancient Greece and Rome and on into the early modern era. Owing to its resemblance to the uterus, birthwort was believed to be useful in childbirth. Many *Aristolochia* species are widely used in Chinese traditional medicine, including *Aristolochia manshuriensis*, which, as Guanmutong, was widely used for the treatment of urinary tract and cardiovascular diseases. Other preparations including *Aristolochia* herbs are used in traditional Chinese medicine to alleviate gastrointestinal symptoms and as antirheumatics, diuretics, and liver tonics.

As is often the case in the history of medicine, it turned out that aristolochic acid had been a topic of considerable interest decades earlier, in a very different context. From the 1950s to the 1970s the National Cancer Institute had conducted a major program to screen plant compounds for antitumor activity. Virtually all the chemotherapeutic agents in use today are the result of that program. In the late 1960s Morris Kupchan, the head of the program, had declared that aristolochic acid was "the most potent antitumor agent" of all the compounds screened. In the late 1970s a German pharmaceutical entrepreneur named Rolf Madaus synthesized the compound in the laboratory and tested it in volunteers in order to study its anti-infection properties, with a view to developing it as a drug.[9] It was, indeed, effective, but then in the early 1980s a German toxicologist showed definitively that aristolochic acid was a carcinogen in rats.[10] At that point Madaus stopped drug development, but his company was able to provide pure aristolochic acid to other researchers.

Prompted by the evidence of carcinogenicity, in the mid-1980s Heinz Schmeiser, a biochemist at the German Cancer Research Center in Heidelberg, demonstrated that aristolochic acid was mutagenic. By 1990 he and his colleagues had published results showing that it could bind to DNA, forming *adducts*, which, if they persist, could lead to the development of cancer.[11] Thus, before the first report about Chinese herbs nephropathy in Belgian women appeared in the *Lancet* in 1993, all the analytic methods for detecting aristolochic acid–DNA adducts had been worked out in Heidelberg.

The two groups of nephrologists—at the Protestant Erasmus Hospital and at the Catholic University of Louvain Hospital—were aware of each other's findings as well as the work of Schmeiser in Heidelberg. Cosyns at Louvain Hospital was first to initiate a collaboration with Schmeiser. The resulting chemical analyses, published in 1996, showed that all renal tissue samples from the Belgian women contained aristolochic acid–DNA adducts and that the cumulative dose of *Aristolochia* was a significant risk factor for kidney disease and urothelial cancer.[12] This provided confirmatory evidence for the substitution of the nephrotoxic and carcinogenic *Aristolochia fangchi* for the benign *Stephania tetranda* and documented exposure in the actual tissues. Vanherweghem and his group also collaborated with Schmeiser, and the landmark *New England Journal of Medicine* paper in 2000 by Nortier and Vanherweghem listed Schmeiser and his colleague as coauthors.[13]

In 2001 the U.S. Food and Drug Administration issued an advisory alerting consumers to immediately discontinue the use of products containing aristolochic acid. Other countries took similar actions. And in 2002 the International Agency for Research on Cancer classified aristolochic acid as "probably carcinogenic to humans."[14]

\* \* \*

It was not until early 2002 that Arthur Grollman, a molecular pharmacologist and head of the Department of Pharmacological Sciences at the School of Medicine at Stony Brook University, came across the *New England Journal of Medicine* article describing the similarity between Chinese herbs nephropathy in the Belgian women and Balkan endemic nephropathy. That linkage immediately "piqued his interest," as he told me when I interviewed him in his office ten years later, and set him on a course of research combining epidemiologic investigations with powerful molecular and genomic techniques. His research would take him to the Balkans and Taiwan and would contribute new insights to our understanding of the mechanisms underlying the development of urothelial cancer and cancer in general. No less important, it would draw attention to a worldwide public health problem.

I knew Arthur from the 1990s when I was in the Department of Preventive Medicine at Stony Brook. As a molecular biologist interested in chemical carcinogenesis, he was always alert to opportunities to study the effects of environmental and occupational exposures on the development of cancer—such as the extensive exposure of workers and residents in the Techa River area in the former Soviet Union to high levels of radiation from a nuclear plant disaster that occurred in the 1950s. For this reason, he has always been eager to collaborate with epidemiologists. On a number of occasions, we had met to discuss possible projects in his office, which showcased striking photographs of his trekking expeditions in the Himalayas.

Today, in his early eighties, Grollman is trim and energetic and totally immersed in his research program. When explaining the intricacies of his work, his manner is low-key and unhurried, and one detects in his speech a trace of his childhood growing up in Texas as the son of an eminent pharmacologist. He smiles benignly as he highlights the twists and turns in the research, the false paths, and the competing claims of different groups. In an age of extreme specialization, he is willing to immerse himself in unfamiliar disciplines and cultures and to learn new technologies in order to pursue a problem that interests him. He has numerous collaborations both within his own institution and with clinicians and scientists in Europe and Asia, and he travels widely to attend meetings and give lectures on his work. His work on the molecular toxicology of aristolochic acid and cancer has become a poster child at the National Institute of Environmental Health Sciences for *translational research*, a term that refers to basic research that can be utilized to develop new treatments.

Grollman has devoted much of his career to studying how specific molecules damage DNA, and the consequences of such damage. Humans—and indeed all animals—have an exquisite system for repairing damage to DNA, and most such damage is repaired. However, when the damage affects key segments of our genetic material—such as tumor suppressor genes or oncogenes—and when the resulting lesions elude repair, this can lead to a mutation that gets perpetuated and eventually develops into a cancer. Tackling the mystery of Balkan nephropathy using the most advanced techniques in molecular genomics would turn out to be the culmination of a career studded with accomplishments. However, Grollman would probably never have gotten involved with this obscure disease if it hadn't been for his interest in an issue that had attracted his attention closer to home.

By the early 2000s Grollman had become aware of the huge and largely unrecognized problem created by the widespread availability of herbal supplements, which had come into vogue in the 1960s and had continued to grow since then. The popularity of these products was reflected in the sales of *Prevention* magazine and the spread of megacompanies like GNC. With the rise of the Internet, their availability and popularity continued to expand. In 2001, $17.8 billion was spent in the United States on dietary supplements, $4.2 billion of it for herbs and other botanicals. Many consumers tend to assume that, because these products are "natural" and are advertised and marketed legally, they must be safe, and that the claims of beneficial effects must have some basis. The reality is quite different. In fact, owing to the growing clout of the dietary and herbal supplements industry, in 1994 Congress had passed the Dietary Supplement Health and Education Act (DSHEA). By defining herbal supplements and botanicals as "dietary supplements," DSHEA exempted them from the more rigorous standards used by the FDA in regulating prescription and over-the-counter drugs and medical devices, essentially leaving it up to the industry to regulate itself.

Soon after DSHEA opened the floodgates for herbal supplements, Grollman and his Baylor College of Medicine colleague Donald Marcus started drawing attention to this alarming state of affairs. Their first effort was to organize a symposium at the national meeting of the Association of

American Medical Colleges. The following year, in 2002, they published an article in the *New England Journal of Medicine* drawing attention to the fact that "natural" is not necessarily safe.[15] Their message was clear and unambiguous: since botanicals are "complex mixtures of chemicals," some of which are potentially toxic, in order to protect the public, these products should be subject to the same rigorous regulation as applies to food and drugs. In 2003, as a case in point, they documented the toxicity of the popular botanical Ma Huang, better known as ephedra, in the journal *Science*.[16] As a result of their writings, Grollman was asked to testify before Congress and the White House Commission on Alternative and Complementary Medicine on the topic of herbal supplements.

As academics, Grollman and Marcus thought that their arguments would carry weight with their colleagues, particularly if they focused on botanicals, which they predicted would have toxicities and little or no reliable evidence of therapeutic value. However, they soon became aware that Complementary and Alternative Medicine, or CAM, and an uncritical attitude toward the use of botanicals were making inroads within the academic community itself. They were taken aback that the deans at prestigious medical schools, including Johns Hopkins, Columbia, Duke, and Harvard, had been persuaded of the value of establishing programs in CAM at their institutions. At Stony Brook in 1997, the dean of the School of Medicine and the director of the University Hospital decided to set up a center for CAM as a way of bringing in funds from this emerging, if academically dubious, discipline. Grollman and several other department heads voiced their opposition to the university's engaging in this area. In spite of their objections, however, the dean hired a pediatrician named Sam Benjamin to head up the new program. When Benjamin gave a lecture, Grollman would attend and ask probing questions, and it got to the point where Benjamin would appear to shrink when he saw Grollman enter the room. By this time, Grollman's annual lecture on pharmacology for the medical students and residents was devoted to a critical examination of the toxicity of botanicals and herbal supplements.[17]

The Stony Brook CAM Center proved to be short-lived and closed down after three years. But because of it, Grollman had become even more aware of what he now saw as a national problem, and he continued to be on the lookout for new material for his lecture and for "ammunition" to expose the facile and dangerous misrepresentations of the purveyors of CAM. It was in this heightened state of alert that in 2002 he came across the *New England Journal of Medicine* article from 2000 by the group from the Erasmus Hospital in Brussels. What piqued Grollman's interest in the article describing Chinese herbs nephropathy in the Belgian women was the likening of the Belgian syndrome to Balkan nephropathy. He had heard about Balkan endemic nephropathy as a medical student at Johns Hopkins, and now he became aware of the long-standing failure to make progress in identifying its cause since it was first recognized forty years earlier.

\* \* \*

In the late 1950s throughout the Balkans (in Bosnia, Serbia, and Croatia, which were then part of the former Yugoslavia, as well as in Romania and Bulgaria), physicians had noticed a mysterious renal disease in certain rural farming villages located along tributaries of the Danube River, the Sava, the Drava, the Morava, and the Kolubara[18] (fig. 6.1). It was documented independently in the different countries, but its features were the same everywhere. The disease was characterized by a unique type of renal

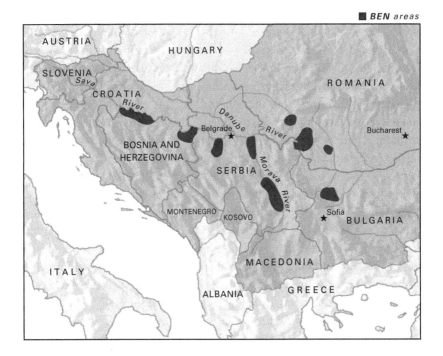

Figure 6.1
Map showing distribution of Balkan endemic nephropathy regions.
*Source*: Maharaj et al. 2014. By permission Springer Publishing Company.

pathology—fibrosis, or scarring, of the renal tubules, progressing invariably to end-stage renal failure. The glomeruli—the capillaries that perform
the first step in filtering the blood—remained untouched until the kidney
was shrunken with fibrosis, so patients didn't show symptoms until the very
late stages of the disease. The geographic distribution of the disease was
also striking. It was limited to rural areas and to families engaged in farming, and it presented a "mosaic pattern"—one village would have it, while
another nearby village did not. Endemic villages were almost always ones
whose fields were located in the floodplain of a river. The disease affected
adults, often in the same household, but never occurred in those less than
18 years of age. The female-to-male ratio was 1.0 or somewhat higher.[19]

Over the next thirty or forty years, clinicians and public health scientists in these countries carried out solid epidemiologic studies with minimal financial support. By conducting surveys of villages—including those
with and without the disease—in defined endemic areas over a number of
decades, researchers were able to describe the distinctive features of the
condition. Because the disease tended to cluster in families, it was logical
to surmise that the condition was hereditary. However, these early epidemiologic investigations pointed strongly to an environmental cause. This
was suggested by the fact that when women in an endemic village who were
not affected moved to an unaffected village, after about fifteen years they
developed the disease. Even more striking was the experience of Ukrainian
migrants who had moved to the endemic area of Croatia at the end of the
nineteenth and beginning of the twentieth centuries. They had been farmers
in Ukraine, and they made up nearly half of the farming population in some
villages in the endemic region. Their way of life was very similar in almost all
respects to that of their Croatian neighbors, except that each group went to
their own churches. Endemic nephropathy did not exist in Ukraine; by the
1950s, however, the migrants had levels of the disease comparable to their
Croatian neighbors. This amounted to what epidemiologists call a "natural
experiment." The fact that two different populations—the indigenous Croats
and the Ukrainian immigrants—both had comparable rates of nephropathy
in the affected areas suggested strongly that the disease was not hereditary
and that some common environmental exposure was involved.[20]

The mysterious condition, which had never appeared anywhere else
in this particular form except in these five countries, was given the ge-
neric appellation of "Balkan endemic nephropathy," or simply "endemic
nephropathy." (Grollman remarked that no people wish to have a disease
associated with their name, and people in the Balkans were delighted

when he and his colleagues eventually showed that this condition was not limited to the Balkans.)

By the 1960s it had also been noticed, first in Bulgaria, that in addition to the occurrence of nephropathy, these same endemic villages had a high incidence of cancer of the upper urinary tract (renal pelvis and ureter), and the cancers frequently occurred in the same patients who had the nephropathy.[21] The vast majority of urothelial cancers worldwide occur in the bladder, with less than 5 percent of tumors involving the upper urinary tract. So it became clear that the unusual form of kidney damage and the rare urothelial cancer of the upper urinary tract associated with it were two features of the same syndrome.

(It is important to clarify that damage to the tubules of the kidney is unrelated to the development of the cancer, which occurs in a different tissue—that which lines the upper urinary tract, which runs from the renal pelvis to the bladder. However, the aristolochic acid–DNA adducts are best measured in the cortex of the kidney because they are concentrated there twentyfold.)

Then in 1964 the World Health Organization organized an international symposium in Dubrovnik at which the different aspects of Balkan nephropathy—clinical, pathological, and epidemiologic—were comprehensively reviewed by scientists from the region and from many other countries as well.[22] Participants considered all the possible explanations, including genetics, viruses, bacteria, immunologic disorders, heavy metals such as lead and cadmium, lignites from coal, and ochratoxin—a fungal toxin. And they could pretty well rule out most of them over the next few years. But the one they eventually focused on was ochratoxin, in part because there were high levels in the blood of the farmers in the villages. In retrospect, it is easy to see that ochratoxin didn't really make sense. The fact is that high levels of the toxin are found in farmers in certain parts of Europe and elsewhere throughout the world, where the incidence of nephropathy is unremarkable. But they chose to overlook that inconvenient fact. Scientists focusing primarily on endemic nephropathy wanted very much to believe that ochratoxin must be involved, and for the next thirty years that was the only theory that got attention.[23]

Actually, an astute Serbian microbiologist named Milenko Ivić had published a paper in 1969 proposing that aristolochic acid toxicity might be responsible for Balkan nephropathy and its associated cancer.[24] Based on his own observations of farming life and unpublished work he had done on aristolochic acid toxicity as a graduate student, Ivić made a compelling argument that all the available facts pointed to contamination of wheat with the seeds of the weed *Aristolochia clematitis*. These facts included the distinctive distribution of the disease (occurring only in villages, never in cities, and often among multiple members of the same household); the plant's renal toxicity, which had also been demonstrated in horses accidentally and experimentally poisoned with *Aristolochia*; and the carcinogenic properties of aristolochic acid, which Ivić himself first demonstrated in rabbits. Other scientists working in the field sometimes cited his paper, but it was always referred to as just another hypothesis. Not one attempt was made to test it, and Professor Ivić died long before Grollman was to prove his hypothesis to be correct.

* * *

Forty years after the initial recognition of Balkan nephropathy, the incidence of the disease had hardly changed. And despite the publication of hundreds of scientific papers and the holding of numerous symposiums, there was no clue as to its cause. This is where things stood in 2002, when Grollman, after reading the article drawing attention to the similarity of Chinese herbs nephropathy to Balkan nephropathy, was seized by the urge to delve into this long-standing unresolved conundrum. The usual way a scientist would go about exploring a new idea would be to apply for a grant from the National Institutes of Health. But this would mean that, even in the best possible case, a year or more would elapse before he could obtain funding, and then, realistically, it would take another two or more years to carry out the study.

Instead, Grollman walked over to his computer and pulled up Google Earth and studied the pattern of the fields and farming villages laid out on either side of the Sava River, several hours east of Zagreb. He had no idea how to go about conducting an epidemiologic study in a remote and unfamiliar region, but it so happened that he and his wife were close friends with a couple from Croatia, the Prelećs. Krsto Preleć was a physicist at Brookhaven National Laboratory, and his wife was a librarian at Stony Brook. They put him in touch with Bojan Jelaković, head of nephrology at the Zagreb University School of Medicine. Thanks to this connection, Grollman was able to arrange a quick visit to Zagreb in the spring of 2002, and Dr. Jelaković, who was to become his main collaborator, drove him to the endemic area. When they got to the village of Kaniža in the focal area of Brodska Posavina, Jelaković said, "Let me show you the black houses." This was the local term for houses that had been abandoned when their owners died of endemic nephropathy. They walked through the village, which had fifty or sixty homes. Several of them were completely run-down, with gaping doors and windows and at least one with the branches of a tree growing through the roof. And Jelaković remarked only half-jokingly that one could determine the local prevalence of nephropathy by counting the number of black houses. Six black houses, 10 percent of the village.

From the endemic village, Jelaković took Grollman to the dialysis clinic at the hospital in Slavonski Brod, the main city in the county. Since the Belgian women had been taking herbs, and since this was a rural area and Grollman knew from his reading that *Aristolochia* had been used as an herb known as "birthwort" for thousands of years in Europe, he had the idea that the patients must have been taking it. With Jelalović acting as translator, he interviewed a number of patients who were tethered to the dialysis machines for up to six hours. The patients were highly cooperative. They and their families were living with the scourge of this inexplicable disease, and they were eager to help anyone who took an interest in it and were comfortable answering probing questions about their way of life. But after interviewing a number of patients, Grollman was convinced that none of them had used any form of herbal medicines. "It was a good idea," he remarked, but it simply didn't fit their medical history.

Grollman's wife had come along on the trip, and they had planned to visit Dubrovnik on the Dalmatian coast. But before they left, he went back to the medical school library in Zagreb, where he happened to know the librarian, who had spent time at Stony Brook as a visiting scholar. She showed him a section of the library that had dust-covered books relating to kidney disease, among which he found a 1956 article from the veterinary school at the university. "Now you would never pick this article up on PubMed, I can tell you," Grollman said. The article, which was in German, described kidney disease in horses, which the authors had linked to their ingesting *Aristolochia clematitis*, a weed that grows in many cultivated fields. Grollman remarked that "the vets knew their subject," having recognized in 1920s that *Aristolochia* plants were toxic for horses. They had published several papers on this topic and had even fed horses *Aristolochia* and studied its toxic effects. "But since these reports were from the veterinary school, their colleagues in the nearby school of medicine didn't pay attention." But what caught Grollman's eye was that the article displayed pictures of fields with *Aristolochia clematitis* growing abundantly. And when he looked at the histopathology of the *Aristolochia*-induced kidney disease in horses, it resembled what was seen in humans. At this point Grollman realized that Balkan nephropathy might have something to do with the wheat used in making bread, which, he had learned on his visit to the endemic region, makes up about 50 or 60 percent of the diet in these poor, rural areas.

Grollman reasoned that the *Aristolochia* had to comingle with the wheat and that it had to be pretty strong to withstand the baking process. He knew that you could pick up evidence of exposure and genetic damage by measuring adducts to aristolochic acid in kidney tissues, as Schmeiser had done in the Belgian women.

To test his hypothesis that aristolochic acid was actually the cause of endemic nephropathy, he asked Jelaković for tissue samples to take back with him. The pathology department in Slavonski Brod had samples stored in formalin, going back forty years, and Jelaković obtained a couple of paraffin-embedded blocks from endemic nephropathy patients, which, after visiting Dubrovnik, Grollman took back to New York. In addition to the age of the samples, they had been whittled down by other investigators who had dug out much of the tissue. In spite of the poor condition of the specimens, Grollman's long-term colleague, Shinya Shibutani, was nevertheless able to tentatively identify aristolactam-DNA adducts using a method he had developed called P32-postlabelling, a type of radioisotope analysis. (This method was a modification of that used to detect aristolochic acid–DNA adducts in tissues from the Belgian women.) But, owing to the treatment of the samples with formaldehyde, the image was blurry, and they could not be 100 percent confident of their conclusion.

Grollman and his collaborators were eager to obtain fresh frozen kidney tissue from patients with endemic nephropathy to confirm their finding, and they got very excited on hearing that two such kidneys were stored frozen in Bulgaria. After lengthy correspondence to get cooperation from the Bulgarian clinicians, they were about to send a collaborator from Croatia to pick up the samples when they learned that the freezer storing the tissues had failed, and the specimens were irrevocably damaged.

Just when he thought all was lost, Grollman was contacted by a malpractice attorney in Providence, Rhode Island. Somehow the attorney had heard about Grollman's work on aristolochic acid, and he told him about a woman who had been given herbs by a local practitioner of alternative medicine. An astute pathologist at the University Hospital in Providence had made the tentative diagnosis of aristolochic acid nephropathy on the woman's biopsy, and he wanted Grollman to confirm it.

Grollman innocently asked whether any of the patient's renal tissue had been saved in pathology and learned that it was standard practice to leave the damaged kidney in place when performing a renal transplant. This particular operation had been performed by a prominent transplant surgeon in Providence. Grollman informed the attorney, and later the transplant surgeon, that it was highly advisable that they operate again to remove the damaged kidneys, since they were very likely to develop urothelial cancer over time. The transplant surgeon agreed, and Grollman was asked about his consultation fee. He replied "none," provided that he would be given access to the fresh frozen tissue when the kidney was received. To make sure he got it, Grollman asked to come to the operating room at the time of the repeat surgery. So on a snowy night in 2003, a few days before Christmas, Grollman flew up to Providence and picked up the kidney personally. (As if to further heighten the drama surrounding this serendipitous acquisition of the crucial tissues, while waiting for his return flight, there was a bomb scare at the airport and the terminal was evacuated. Grollman was worried that airport security would not allow him through with his samples marked "Biohazard—Biological Materials." However, his explanation was accepted and he caught his flight.) It was this fresh kidney tissue that he used to definitively identify aristolactam-DNA adducts, as described in a landmark paper in the *Proceedings of the National Academy of Sciences* (2007).[25]

While Grollman and his colleagues were refining their methods for detecting aristolochic acid-adducts, by coincidence Tjaša Hranjec, a Stony Brook medical student who was fluent in Serbo-Croatian, came to him looking for a summer research project. Under his supervision (through frequent telephone calls and e-mails) and with assistance from Dr. Jelaković, Tjaša provided the "boots on the ground" necessary to carry out an initial case-control study of Balkan endemic nephropathy in the endemic region of Croatia. She conducted interviews with patients and controls, obtained all the needed specimens, and helped solve the logistical problems that arose. She met with the patients Grollman had interviewed in the dialysis clinic, including a farmer who took her out to his fields. It was after the harvest, and she saw *Aristolochia clematitis* growing scattered throughout the wheat fields, just the way the horse paper had described fifty years earlier. The seeds come to fruition at the height of the summer, and the farmers use very primitive methods—little beyond the scythe—to harvest the wheat. She asked the farmer why he didn't get rid of this weed. And he said, "Doc, it's very hot out here, and it's not gonna do you any harm. Look at all the weeds."[26]

While in the endemic area, Tjaša had visited a retired miller and his old-fashioned mill that local farmers had used for generations. After harvesting the wheat each year, farmers would take it back to their homes and store it in the attic. Every two weeks they would take grain to the miller, have it ground, give the miller 10 percent in payment, and bring the flour home.

The women would then bake five-pound loaves of bread. The first week the bread would be fresh, but by the second week, it would be stale and they would feed it to the animals. But bread constituted 50 percent of the farm diet. And the aristolochic acid in the seeds is very stable and therefore survives the temperature of the baking oven.

The initial study included twenty-eight cases who met the criteria for endemic nephropathy, thirty individuals with other forms of renal disease, and thirty healthy controls. Using a detailed questionnaire, the researchers collected information on demographics, exposure to potentially toxic substances, diet, agricultural practices, and other factors that might contribute to endemic nephropathy. In addition, seeds of *Aristolochia clematitis*, obtained from plants growing in the endemic region, were analyzed for their aristolochic acid content.

The results of this initial epidemiologic study showed that twenty to thirty years earlier, patients with endemic nephropathy had encountered *Aristolochia clematitis* in the fields much more frequently than controls did. All groups reported that since that time there had been a significant increase in the use of herbicides, leading to a reduction in the prevalence of the weed in recent years. Chemical analysis established that the seeds of *A. clematitis* contained 0.65 percent aristolochic acid and that it was likely that the seeds had mingled with the wheat grain during harvesting. The results were published in the *Croatian Medical Journal* in order to get the word out quickly to clinicians in Balkan countries who were taking care of endemic nephropathy patients.[27]

Now Grollman had a hypothesis. Ingestion of aristolochic acid combined with individual susceptibility accounts for all the epidemiologic and clinical features of endemic nephropathy. And the hypothesis had a corollary: Balkan endemic nephropathy, Chinese herbs nephropathy, and aristolochic acid nephropathy were one and the same disease. Or, in Grollman's notation: BEN = CHN = AAN.

* * *

Grollman was undertaking his study in Croatia just after the end of the wars among Balkan countries with their widespread atrocities, and he remarked on the geopolitics he and Dr. Jelaković had to contend with. "The five physician groups who had studied this rarely talked to each other, even when three of them were part of one country—Yugoslavia—much less collaborate on medical research." He knew that—in a perverse reflection of nationalism—they would all say that "their" disease was different. He realized that, if they were going to solve the riddle of Balkan endemic nephropathy, they were going to have to work together. It took a good deal of informal diplomacy to succeed in getting tissue samples from Serbia, Bosnia, and Croatia. In addition to the political animosities, Grollman and his collaborators had to overcome distrust on the part of some clinicians and deal with very different medical practices. For example, he needed tissue specimens from the cancer patients to analyze for DNA adducts and mutations. But when he asked for biopsy specimens, he learned that the nephrologists did not perform biopsies on patients with suspected endemic nephropathy. Nor did they any longer perform autopsies on patients dying of the disease. It looked like he was never going to get the kidney samples he needed for a systematic analysis of adducts in human kidneys. But then he realized that the urothelium extends into the kidney pelvis and it's a curable cancer—the surgeon removes the affected kidney, so he could get both tissues into the bargain. The urologists were doing two or three operations per month. So he asked, "What happens to the kidney?" "Oh, we throw that away." He told them, "Please don't throw it away anymore." Since the cancer was so common in this area, all one had to do was get the cooperation of the urologists who did the surgery in Slavonski Brod and the pathologist, who were pleased to provide the samples. So he got both the kidneys and the urothelium at the same time.

Encouraged by these developments, Grollman and colleagues went on to conduct molecular studies of upper urothelial cancer including cases from endemic areas in Bosnia and Serbia, as well as Croatia, and using patients with upper urinary tract cancers from nonendemic areas as controls. They detected adducts to aristolochic acid in 85 percent of nonsmoking patients with nephropathy and upper urothelial cancer living in endemic regions. These adducts persist in the renal cortex for decades, making it likely that people with the exposure would eventually develop cancer. Significantly, adducts were not detected in patients with upper urinary tract cancer living in Zagreb or Belgrade. The investigators concluded that aristolochic acid–DNA adducts provide a robust "biomarker" of exposure to aristolochic acid.[28]

The comparison between the effects of exposure to aristolochic acid in the Brussels weight-loss spa and those of long-term dietary exposure in the Balkans was instructive. On average the women in Brussels were exposed to their regimen for twenty months, and progression to end-stage renal disease also occurred within months. In the Balkans, where both men and women were affected, lower-dose exposure to the aristolochic acid–contaminated bread had occurred over decades, and the average age of onset of nephropathy occurred in the fourth or fifth decade of life. The Belgian women developed upper urothelial cancer within two to six years following the end of their exposure, in contrast to a much longer interval in the Balkans, ranging from twenty to thirty years and roughly ten years after the onset of nephropathy. To a large extent, these differences were likely due to the fact that the Belgian women ingested a much higher dose of aristolochic acid over a short period of time, whereas in the Balkans the typical dose of aristolochic acid was about one-tenth that of the Belgian women, and typically exposure extended from childhood over the better part of a lifetime.[29] Regarding the potency of *Aristolochia*, Grollman commented that ten seeds of *Aristolochia* scattered among perhaps ten thousand seeds of wheat in a loaf of homemade bread was enough to cause disease. The fact that aristolochic acid is both a kidney toxin and a carcinogen, together with the persistence of the damage over a lifetime, make it stand out among environmental mutagens.

The much shorter "induction period" for nephropathy among the Belgian women and the fact that they had all attended the same clinic allowed alert clinicians to quickly pinpoint Chinese herbs as the probable cause, whereas in the Balkans, owing to the chronic exposure to a lower dose, the disease developed slowly and insidiously, and it took forty years to identify the causative exposure.

\* \* \*

The presence of DNA adducts to aristolochic acid in tissues from patients with upper urothelial cancers who were long-term residents of endemic areas suggested that aristolochic acid–induced mutations might play a role in causing the cancer. However, the nature of the damage and how it led to the development of cancer were unclear. Grollman and colleagues proceeded to make a novel contribution to understanding the mechanism by which aristolochic acid induces upper urothelial cancer.

Over the past thirty years discoveries in molecular biology have transformed our understanding of how cancer develops. This new understanding can be stated simply: cancer is a genetic disease. Every individual has a unique genetic identity inscribed in the DNA in every cell in his or her body. Within the DNA, segments of four nucleic acids, or "bases," specify every protein that is made and every physiologic process. The four bases are adenine, guanine, thymine, and cytosine (A, G, T, C). Errors in DNA occur routinely, but most are corrected thanks to our exquisite "copyediting" machinery. If, however, a change in single nucleic acid base in a key gene eludes repair, this can lead to the development of cancer. It is now believed that a handful of mutations to key genes drive the complex, multifactorial, multistep carcinogenic process. Among the most important events are the inactivation of tumor suppressor genes and the activation of oncogenes. Mutations in these genes may be caused by physical agents (e.g., ultraviolet radiation, X-rays), chemical agents (such as benzene, arsenic, benzo(a)pyrene, and vinyl chloride), viruses, and bacteria, or may be inherited. p53 is a major tumor suppressor gene, which is often referred to as part of the "braking system" that protects against cancer. Mutations of the p53 gene are present in roughly 50 percent of all human cancers and occur in different locations along the gene.

Roughly twenty years ago, the discovery of so-called signature or fingerprint mutations had caused great excitement among cancer researchers. This referred to alterations in the sequence of nucleic acid bases in the p53 gene that could serve as a marker of exposure to a specific agent, which plays a role in the induction of a specific type of cancer.[30] Bert Vogelstein, a leading figure in the field of carcinogenesis, at Johns Hopkins, was coauthor on the first paper that made a strong case for a signature mutation in the p53 gene specifically associated with exposure to aflatoxin, a chemical produced by a fungus that grows on peanuts and corn in southern Africa and China, and that plays a role in primary cancer of the liver in those regions. This work generated enormous enthusiasm for the identification of other signature mutations associated with other carcinogenic exposures. However, few comparable fingerprint mutations have been identified in the past twenty years.

The fact that mutations in p53 are also present in about 50 percent of upper urothelial cancers led Grollman and colleagues to examine specific mutations in tissues from patients with endemic nephropathy who had developed upper urothelial cancer. Performing genomic analysis, they identified a unique signature mutation in p53, involving the substitution of thymine for adenine, referred to as an "A T transversion."[31] (Changes of this type have particularly drastic effects because they involve a dramatic change in the chemical structure of DNA.) They also showed that, owing to its location on the nontranscribed stand of the p53 gene, this change eluded repair. This clarified at the molecular level why these adducts persist for decades and eventually lead to cancer. More recent work has shown that the overall mutation rate in aristolochic acid–associated cancers is several times higher than that caused by other carcinogens, such as tobacco and ultraviolet light.

By 2007 the International Agency for Research on Cancer in Lyon had compiled a worldwide databank of genetic sequences of different cancers

that researchers can consult.[32] When Grollman compared the p53 mutation pattern in patients with upper urothelial cancer from endemic areas
with that of all urothelial cancer cases worldwide in the IARC databank,
78 percent of the former had the A → T transversion compared to only
5 percent of the twenty-five thousand urothelial cancers in the databank. If
one limits the comparison to upper urothelial cancers in the IARC database,
less than 1 percent have the A → T transversion. As Grollman put it, "So, the
game's over right there. This mutation clearly is dominant and a signature of
aristolochic acid–associated upper urothelial cancer." What this means is that
the way in which aristolochic acid induces cancer is distinct from the way in
which other agents such as tobacco, aflatoxin, or X-rays induce cancer. According to Grollman, after aflatoxin, this is the first truly distinctive signature
associated with a major chemical exposure to be identified in many years.

With this work that was published in the *Proceedings of the National
Academy of Sciences USA* in 2007, Grollman and colleagues had confirmed their predictions. Seeds of *A. clematitis* comingle with the wheat
grain used to prepare home-baked bread. Aristolochic acid–DNA adducts are present in the renal cortex and in urothelial tumor tissue of
patients with Balkan endemic nephropathy. And finally, a single, specific
signature mutation is the most common p53 mutation in upper urothelial cancer associated with endemic nephropathy. They had demonstrated
that BEN = CHN = AAN.[33]

When the results of the study in the Balkans were complete, each national group of collaborators had to organize a separate symposium—one
in Zagreb, one in Belgrade, and one in Sarajevo—for Grollman to present
the work before physicians and researchers from each Balkan country were
willing to accept that "we had proved that something other than ochratoxin
was responsible for Balkan endemic nephropathy."

\* \* \*

After working out the mechanism by which aristolochic acid modifies
DNA and identifying the unique mutational signature in the p53 gene present in the majority of aristolochic acid–associated upper urothelial cancers,
Grollman saw that another critical question needed to be answered. In spite
of the strong link between ingestion of aristolochic acid, whether in powdered Chinese herbs or in bread contaminated with seeds from *Aristolochia clematitis*, not everyone who was exposed became ill. In Belgium, 105
women developed nephropathy out of 1,800 who were exposed, or about

5 percent. And in endemic villages in Croatia, 5–10 percent of residents of these villages develop endemic nephropathy. This suggested that genetic susceptibility, or resistance, to the effects of aristolochic acid influenced one's risk of developing the disease. In laboratory experiments with mice, Rosenquist and Grollman had confirmed the existence of genes governing susceptibility or resistance to aristolochic acid–induced nephropathy. Thus an important question that remains to be answered is, what is the genetic basis for human sensitivity to aristolochic acid?

Over the past three decades a major thrust of biomedical research has been to identify the genes and genetic variants that make someone either susceptible or resistant to chronic disease, including cancer. During this period, at an ever-increasing rate, scientists had been examining "candidate genes" suspected of playing a role in susceptibility to specific diseases. When the rough version of the human genome was announced in 2000 and featured on the covers of *Nature* and *Science*, this search for candidate genes only intensified. Grollman pointed out to me that "if you look back, during the years before 2007, hundreds of papers were published in leading journals saying, 'We found this gene that contributes to susceptibility.' But if you ask, 'Which studies were replicated?' the answer is: very few—perhaps only one or two each year! Everyone had their favorite gene, but no one did the statistics to remind themselves that there are 23,000 genes, so you are going to get a lot of false positives."

In 2007 the field moved away from the approach of looking for hypothesis-driven candidate genes and embraced "genome-wide association studies" in which whole genome sequences are compared between those with a disease and those without. Large sample sizes are required for these studies—thousands or tens of thousands of patients—and the requirement for replication of results is built into the new approach. As Grollman put it, "genome-wide, non-hypothesis testing trumps candidate genes." By the time Grollman turned to the question of susceptibility in 2009, the methods for sequencing whole genomes and identifying all potentially relevant genes had been fundamentally transformed, and so-called "next-generation sequencing" had become possible.

Grollman is collaborating with Bert Vogelstein and Ken Kinzler at Johns Hopkins, using advanced DNA sequencing techniques to identify genes that influence a person's risk of developing upper urothelial cancer, given exposure to aristolochic acid. This new work has revealed that exposure to aristolochic acid is associated with a number of somatic mutations throughout the genome, in addition to the ones in TP53. Nearly three-quarters of these mutations exhibit the distinctive signature A → T transversions. The pattern of mutations in aristolochic acid–associated upper urothelial cancer contrasts starkly with that seen in smoking-associated upper urothelial cancer cases.[34]

\* \* \*

The outbreak of Chinese herbs nephropathy in Brussels resulted from the unfortunate substitution of one Chinese herb for another. And Balkan endemic nephropathy proved to be a long-standing environmental disease due to the unrecognized presence of the toxic weed *Aristolochia clematitis* growing in the local wheat fields, which led to contamination of the grain used in preparing homemade bread. But it now became clear to Grollman that the potential impact of the toxic and carcinogenic effects of *Aristolochia* was likely to be much greater than suggested by these two localized episodes, since in various forms this herb has been used on virtually every continent going back thousands of years. It now occurred to him that *Aristolochia*-caused nephropathy and cancer might be global diseases.

When he looked for reported cases of *Aristolochia*-associated upper urothelial cancer, however, there were no systematically recorded statistics. All he found were small numbers based on recent case reports: 4 in both the United Kingdom and France, 1 in both Spain and Germany, 128 in Belgium, 1 in South Korea, 6 in Japan, 33 in Taiwan, and 116 in China. These were individual cases where there was some indication that the person had used Chinese herbs, but there was no objective evidence of exposure, such as aristolochic acid–DNA adducts. Grollman realized that his two biomarkers—for aristolochic acid–DNA adducts and for the signature mutation—provided a robust means of determining the prevalence of aristolochic acid–induced urothelial cancer in different populations with a high degree of accuracy.

Aware that Taiwan had the highest incidence of upper urothelial cancer, as well as one of the highest rates of kidney disease in the world, Grollman contacted urologists at the National University Hospital in Taipei and suggested that *Aristolochia* might be a contributing factor. The urologists were skeptical, but they agreed to collaborate. In 2010 a group of Taiwanese researchers had published the results of a countrywide case-control study of Chinese herbal products containing aristolochic acid and risk of urinary tract cancer.[35] Owing to the existence of a national health insurance system that covers 96 percent of the Taiwanese population, they were able to access all prescriptions for Chinese herbs filled between January 1, 1997, and December 31, 2002. Comparing the prescription histories of nearly 4,600 urinary tract cancer cases enrolled during a one-year period to those of 174,701 controls, the authors showed that the risk of urinary tract cancer increased in a dose-dependent manner with increasing intake of Chinese herbs containing aristolochic acid. The scale of use of herbal supplements—and their potential impact on kidney disease and urinary tract cancer—was driven home by a systematic analysis of prescriptions filled by a 200,000-person random sample of the entire insured population of Taiwan between 1997 and 2003. Approximately one-third of the sample consumed herbs containing, or likely to contain, aristolochic acid. Approximately 140,000 pounds of one of these herbs, *Aristolochia debilis* (Quing-Muxiang), are imported annually into Taiwan.

Grollman proceeded to carry out a molecular epidemiologic study to learn whether exposure to aristolochic acid, found in all *Aristolochia* herbal remedies, contributed to the high incidence of upper urothelial cancer in Taiwan. The study design was similar to that used in the Balkans. The study included 151 patients with upper urothelial cancer and 25 patients with renal cell cancer (the most common type of kidney cancer) serving as a control group. Both groups were equally exposed to the toxin, based on the presence of aristolochic acid–DNA adducts. However, similar to the results in the Balkans, the pattern of p53 mutational spectra in Taiwanese patients with upper urothelial cancer showed a predominance of the rare A → T transversions, whereas this mutation was absent in the controls. Furthermore, the combination of aristolochic acid–DNA adducts and presence of the signature mutation underscored the close association between exposure to aristolochic acid and its carcinogenic effect. These results were published in *Proceedings of the National Academy of Sciences* in April 2012, shortly before I visited Grollman, and they had generated interest in the scientific community as well as millions of hits on the Internet, particularly in Asia.[36]

As Grollman put it, describing the p53 mutation results from the Balkans and those from Taiwan, "when you put them side-by-side, they're almost mirror images. The important thing is to compare the two. When you look at those mutations in a single base pair in DNA—in the Balkans and Taiwan—they go absolutely on top of each other. It's not even one base off. You have different ethnic groups, different environments, and different routes of exposure. To have that degree of specificity—that is solid evidence for the global nature of this disease."

In addition, the researchers noted that the prevalence of adducts and of the signature mutation was slightly higher in female compared to male cases, and women in Taiwan are more likely than men to obtain prescriptions for herbal supplements. Thus the higher incidence of upper urothelial cancer among Taiwanese women may reflect, in part, their more extensive exposure to *Aristolochia*-containing herbal remedies.

\* \* \*

Referring to the hundred-plus case reports of *Aristolochia*-induced upper urothelial cancer in all of China, Grollman said, "A hundred cases! Either the Han Chinese in China have different genes—which seems very unlikely—or they are not recognizing or reporting it." *Aristolochia* has been used as an herbal remedy in China since at least the Han dynasty, two thousand years ago. In the 1500s the Chinese herbalist Li Shizen assembled all previous *materia medica* from China, which included various herbs in the *Aristolochia* family. This was around the time of Paracelsus in Europe, who, by the way, also used *Aristolochia*, where it was known as "birthwort." But whereas Western medicine has advanced dramatically since Paracelsus, discarding his remedies, Li Shizen's herbal compendium was still being used until recently as a primary reference by schools of Chinese Traditional Medicine. Grollman remarked, "It's important in terms of the Chinese cultural traditions to realize that everything that needed to be known about Chinese traditional medicine practiced today was known hundreds of years ago." If you use herbal medicine in China, Li Shizen is still a preeminent authority to consult, just as we would go to Goodman and Gilman's indispensable *The Pharmacological Basis of Therapeutics*, now in its twelfth edition.

In presenting data from Taiwan, Grollman and his Taiwanese collaborators reported that the incidence of upper urothelial cancer in Taiwan had increased about fourfold from 1983 to 2007, whereas its incidence in other countries had remained at the same level over this time period. How was one to explain the sharp increase in the incidence of the cancer in Taiwan, if, in fact, use of *Aristolochia*-containing Chinese herbs had been an important factor all along? By examining the production and use of *Aristolochia* herbs in China, particularly since the 1930s, the authors were able to correlate the progressive increase in upper urothelial cancer with the systematic replacement of traditionally used Mutong herbs with *Aristolochia manchuriensis*. In mainland China, this practice appears to have begun in the 1930s, when, owing to the Japanese occupation, the usual sources of Mutong in southern provinces were cut off. The practice had become widespread by the 1950s and continued until 2003, when these substitutions were outlawed by the Chinese government. The presence of aristolochic acid in *A. manchuriensis* exported from China to Taiwan between 1995 and 2003, as well as to other Asian countries, Great Britain, and the Netherlands, has been documented by chemical analyses. Thus, assuming a latency period of thirty years, the carcinogenic effects of aristolochic acid would be expected to have become increasingly manifest in Taiwan starting in the mid-1980s, as in fact they are.

The concluding sentence in the *PNAS* paper in 2012 delivered a sobering message regarding the implications for the future. Given the "the lifelong persistence" of the aristolochic acid–DNA adducts in target tissues and the "irreversible damage to the proximal . . . renal tubules caused by aristolochic acid, persons treated with *Aristolochia* herbal preparations at any time in their life are at significant risk of developing upper urothelial carcinoma and/or chronic renal disease, thereby creating an international public health problem of considerable magnitude."[37]

Since the traditional practice of Chinese herbal medicine in Taiwan mirrors that in China and other Asian countries, Grollman surmised that upper urothelial cancer and its attendant aristolochic acid nephropathy must also be prevalent in these countries where *Aristolochia* herbs have long been widely used for the treatment and prevention of disease. But when he contacted clinicians in China, he quickly became aware of the psychology and culture surrounding the use of traditional Chinese herbs. Many clinicians were reluctant to discuss the issue. In China, the government controls the distribution of traditional herbs, and people don't want to be seen criticizing the government—or traditional Chinese medicine. At a nephrology meeting, he encountered the head of nephrology at a major hospital that treats patients with *Aristolochia* poisoning. This individual confirmed that several *Aristolochia* herbs were still listed in the Chinese pharmacopeia—twelve years after the first report about the women in Belgium and two years after the Chinese government had outlawed the use of most *Aristolochia* herbs. Grollman asked what was being done in the way of public health measures to prevent the now well-documented consequences of exposure to the herbs: "You know it, I know it, the world knows it." The nephrologist replied, "All I can do is take care of my patients."

A number of Chinese nationals with kidney disease deduced that they had been poisoned by *Aristolochia* plants, and they reasoned that, if the government controls industry, the government should be responsible for their adverse effects. In fact, a class-action suit—apparently the first in

Chinese history—was brought against the government in 2004.[38] However, other than a single article in the *China Times* nothing more has been heard about the case.

The large herb company based in Hong Kong, Tong Ren Tang, sells herbs not only in China but elsewhere in Asia and throughout the world. In 2003 the Chinese government banned the use of *Aristolochia* herbs in the popular product Longdan Xiegan Wan, although it continued to be marketed under the same name. Grollman analyzed samples of Longdan Xiegan Wan before and after the ban, and he could see the aristolochic acid content of this product had disappeared. Since one manufacturer dominated the market for industrially produced herbals, the government was able to stop exposure to aristolochic acid in the form of Longdan Xiegan Wan. As he noted, however, several other forms of *Aristolochia*, including the toxic and carcinogenic varieties, are still listed in the official pharmacopeia, and throughout China it is relatively easy to obtain them. Furthermore, as of 2003, more than one hundred *Aristolochia* products were still available on the Internet.[39]

Data on production of *Aristolochia* species in China are available, and in one report, the amount produced was enough to cause toxic effects in one hundred million people. As Grollman commented, "There is nothing else you use medicinal herbs for, so, unless they discarded it, which seems very unlikely—by a conservative estimate, approximately one hundred million people in China and elsewhere have been exposed to the toxin, and those that are susceptible are at risk of developing aristolochic acid–induced upper urothelial carcinoma and chronic kidney disease."

After encountering bureaucratic resistance, Grollman finally succeeded in initiating a collaborative study of upper urothelial tract cancer at the Shanghai Cancer Hospital. As expected, the great majority of patients with upper urothelial cancer (over 85 percent) showed evidence of exposure to aristolochic acid in the form of adducts and the signature mutation.[40]

The latest development in the unfolding story of aristolochic acid–associated cancer entails new work from Europe and Asia suggesting that aristolochic acid–induced carcinogenesis may not be limited to upper urothelial cancer but may play a role in some liver cancers and renal cell cancer (the most common type of kidney cancer).[41]

\* \* \*

It was only due to the fortuitous presentation of multiple women from the same weight loss spa at clinics in Brussels that the harmful effects of

*Aristolochia* came to light. The discovery of a cluster of young women with kidney fibrosis set in motion a twenty-year research effort that has shed new light on Balkan nephropathy, the mechanisms of cancer causation, and a serious international public health problem. Had it not been for the concentration of exposed women with similar pathology in a single city, the effects of *Aristolochia* might well have gone unnoticed. What does this mean for people in the United States? This takes us back to the short-lived program at Stony Brook devoted to Complementary and Alternative Medicine.

Today Americans spend more than $32 billion a year on different combinations of vitamins, minerals, botanicals, probiotics, amino acids, and other supplement ingredients, and more than half of American adults use these products.[42] Herbal supplements account for roughly one-fifth of the total. A majority of consumers believe, wrongly, that the government requires manufacturers to report all adverse effects and that the FDA must approve supplements before they are sold.[43] Few consumers of supplements are aware of the implications of the Dietary Supplements and Health Education Act, which was passed by Congress in 1994 with strong support from the supplements industry and its political allies. By defining herbal supplements and botanicals as "dietary supplements," DSHEA excluded them from the more rigorous standards used in regulating prescription, and even over-the-counter, drugs. Unlike prescription drugs, supplements do not have to undergo premarket testing before they can be sold to consumers. Rather, they are assumed to be safe based until proven otherwise. The FDA has the unrealistic charge of identifying and recalling dangerous supplements only after they have caused harm.[44]

Since DSHEA was enacted, the number of dietary supplements on the market has surged from roughly four thousand to more than fifty-five thousand.[45] However, of the fifty-one thousand products introduced since 1994, only 170 (0.3 percent) have any documentation of their safety.[46] Major deficiencies in the oversight of dietary supplements include the lack of standardization to guard against adulteration and to ensure a consistent level of the active ingredients;[47] adverse interactions between herbal supplements and prescribed drugs, including chemotherapy; the absence of premarketing testing for safety, as is required for prescription and over-the-counter drugs; deceptive marketing by producers of dietary supplements and lack of adequate labeling to inform consumers about the nature and regulation of these products; and the failure to require reporting of all adverse effects promptly to the FDA.[48]

Owing to the lack of a proper surveillance system for reporting adverse events promptly and directly to the FDA, harm from supplements is seriously underreported, and in a number of cases the FDA has been woefully slow to act. According to Marcus and Grollman, "It took the agency more than ten years to remove from the market ephedra-containing herbal weight-loss products that had caused hundreds of deaths and thousands of adverse events."[49] More recently, in 2011, the Department of Defense banned supplements containing the stimulant DMAA from military bases because of safety concerns, but it took the FDA an additional sixteen months to alert consumers about DMAA's risks, and despite the agency's efforts the stimulant is still present in dozens of supplements.[50]

In the most recent manifestation of the dangers of inadequate oversight of dietary supplements, as of March 2014, the Centers for Disease Control and Prevention have documented an outbreak of hepatitis involving ninety-seven cases and one death in sixteen states linked to the "fat-burning" sports supplement OxyElitePro.[51] Most of the cases were adolescents, and roughly half occurred in Hawaii, where, in 2015, local officials reported one death and two liver transplants. The effects of OxyElitePro were picked up only because of an alert transplant surgeon in Hawaii.[52]

An example of a more systematic effort to gauge the extent of adverse events linked to use of supplements is the Drug-Induced Liver Injury Network, which includes eight U.S. referral centers.[53] Between 2004 and 2013 patients presenting with liver damage at these centers were evaluated for use of medications and herbal and dietary supplements and were followed to ascertain outcomes, including deaths and transplantations. Sixteen percent of all cases of liver damage were attributed to supplements. The most commonly used products implicated were bodybuilding supplements. During the ten-year period the frequency of liver injury caused by supplements increased from 7 percent to 20 percent. This one effort—focused on only one of many types of harm—represents only a first step in documenting the effects of supplements.

A recent study used nationally representative surveillance data from sixty-three emergency departments from 2004 through 2013 to estimate the number of visits because of adverse events related to dietary supplements.[54] The authors estimated that 23,000 emergency department visits in the United States every year were attributable to adverse events involving dietary supplements. The most common problems were cardiac symptoms from weight-loss or energy products among young adults and swallowing problems, often associated with micronutrients, among older adults.

Manufacturers of dietary supplements, their trade associations, and their political supporters in Congress claim that the industry is being unfairly branded owing to the misconduct of a small number of supplement producers. However, this position reflects either cynicism motivated by self-interest—the supplements industry is hugely profitable—or an ideological opposition to tighter regulation, or both. Opponents of tighter oversight of supplements rely on the fundamental confusions and misunderstandings that are widespread regarding these products. First, documented harm and the potential for harm from supplements need to be balanced against the benefits conferred by these products. In spite of claims that are made for a wide range of beneficial effects, in the majority of cases in which popular supplements have been evaluated in clinical trials, no evidence of a benefit was found.[55] Second, while many supplements may indeed be harmless, even if a small percentage of the fifty-five thousand products on the market pose a risk of serious harm, this could affect thousands of consumers.[56]

It should be clear from the record that the problem goes much deeper than the malfeasance of a few rogue supplement manufacturers and that the stakes are not trivial. Those who argue that the current system is adequate to protect consumers should remember that people failed to recognize the nephrotoxic effects of *Aristolochia* in spite of its use in many cultures worldwide over thousands of years. In my interview with him, Grollman explained why: "The reason, of course, is quite simple. It's painless, and the damage happens much later, so you don't put together the fact that you took this medicine and ten years later, you have kidney failure. It's been part of Ayurvedic, European, Chinese, and South American medicine for centuries. All of the great civilizations have used it. And not one reported its toxicity until the Belgians did twenty years ago. There are certain things that tradition can't tell you."

Commenting on the disturbing lack of oversight and regulation of these poorly studied herbal products, many of which have known toxicities, Grollman referred to the thalidomide episode in the 1950s in Europe and to the Belgian women: "The next time we may not be lucky enough to have observations on women from a Brussels spa to alert us to a danger." His take-home message: "DSHEA needs to be amended, and it needs to be amended fast."

# 7

# HPV, Cancer, and Beyond
## *The Anatomy of a Triumph*

The stupidest virus is cleverer than the cleverest immunologist.
—GEORGE KLEIN

In the past two decades it has become clear that infection with certain viruses—as well as certain bacteria—accounts for a substantial proportion of cancer worldwide. However, this knowledge has been achieved only with great difficulty and after pursuing many false leads. The question of the possible role of infection in the cancer process was first raised in 1911 when Peyton Rous of the Rockefeller Institute in New York succeeded in inducing tumors in healthy chickens by injecting them with chicken sarcoma virus from tumor-bearing chickens.[1] But owing to the difficulty of demonstrating the causal role of a virus in human cancer—a disease that often takes decades to develop—it would be another fifty years before there was compelling evidence for a direct link between a virus and a specific cancer in humans. When this evidence finally emerged, it came from a remote corner of the world and was due to the acuity and persistence of a general surgeon working in colonial Africa.

After the end of World War II the Irish physician-surgeon and Presbyterian missionary Denis Parsons Burkitt went to Uganda to minister to people with virtually no access to medical care. In 1957 he was asked to see a 5-year-old boy whose face was deformed by a swollen jaw. Soon after he saw a girl with identical swelling of the jaw and noticed that as the disease progressed she developed swelling in other organs as well.[2] This led him to undertake a meticulous search of district medical records, which revealed that rapidly growing tumors of the jaw were common in children in Uganda and were often associated with tumors in other parts of the body. Tumors of the jaw were, in fact, the most common childhood cancer in Africa as well as the fastest-growing childhood tumor. While the common occurrence of this tumor in African children had been noted early in the twentieth century, Burkitt was the first to posit that the apparently different childhood cancers were all manifestations of a "single distinctive tumour syndrome."[3] Two years after his initial publication in 1958, two of his colleagues identified the tumor as a lymphoma. Although Burkitt himself continued to refer to the "African lymphoma," the newly identified cancer came to be known as "Burkitt's lymphoma."[4]

To trace the contours of the disease, Burkitt first sent an illustrated leaflet and questionnaire to medical practitioners throughout Africa. (The printing and postage costs were covered by a £25 sterling grant from the British government.) To maximize the accuracy of reporting, he hit on the idea of using the distinctive swelling of the jaw in young children as an "index" of the disease, since any medical practitioner who had seen a case was unlikely to forget it or to mistake it for any other condition. The responses to his questionnaire indicated that the tumor occurred in a belt across Central Africa. To obtain a finer-grained picture of what distinguished areas where the tumor was prevalent from those where it was absent, Burkitt and two physician friends organized a "tumor safari," whose purpose was, in his words, "to determine more accurately the limits of this 'tumor belt' and the physical and climatic conditions determining the boundaries."[5] In an inspired formulation that likened the task of tracing the geographical boundaries of the occurrence of the tumor to the surgeon's task of delineating the boundaries of a cancerous lesion, Burkitt referred to his journeys as "surgical biopsies" in which the pathologist attempts to define the "edges" that separate diseased from normal tissue.

In the course of a ten-week safari, the three friends covered ten thousand miles and visited fifty-six hospitals in nine countries. In a paper in the *British Medical Journal* in 1962, Burkitt gave a methodical description of their findings and included four maps displaying the data in different ways. Their surveys showed that the "lymphoma belt" stretched across equatorial Africa extending roughly 15° on either side of the equator and continued south in a "tail" along the east coast. The tumor was prevalent in areas at lower altitude and with greater rainfall and was often concentrated along rivers. The greater the distance from the equator, the lower the upper limit

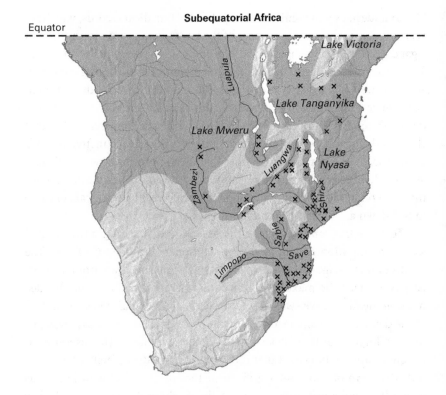

**Figure 7.1**
Map of subequatorial Africa showing areas with Burkitt's lymphoma.
*Source*: Burkitt 1962. By permission BMJ.

on the altitude at which the tumor occurred. Burkitt noted that because of climatic and topographic differences, the tumor could be prevalent in one area and absent in another area less than one hundred miles away. As a number of his colleagues pointed out, the epidemiological maps of malaria and the tumor belt overlapped.

Based on his findings, Burkitt concluded that the effect of altitude must reflect the requirement of a minimum temperature of 60 degrees Fahrenheit. And he went on to speculate that "the fact that this unusual tumor is temperature dependent, implies that some vector may be involved in its transmission. This in turn suggests the possibility that a virus is implicated."[6]

On a visit to London in March 1961, Burkitt presented the results of his research in a lecture entitled "The Commonest Children's Cancer in Tropical Africa—A Hitherto Unrecognised Syndrome." At the back of the lecture hall was a young pathologist named Anthony Epstein of the Bland Sutton Institute. Epstein was working on the role of viruses in carcinogenesis, and he had been drawn by the title of the lecture. He later recalled that he was riveted by Burkitt's description of the tumor's geographical distribution as well as by its association with different organs within the body: "I could hardly sit still because it was immediately clear that anything which had its distribution determined by temperature and rainfall had a biological cause. And of course for me working with the Rous sarcoma virus, a tumor virus of animals, it had to be that it was a virus induced tumor in humans, and that so far as I was concerned was it."[7] The two men spoke after the lecture, and Burkitt agreed to send Epstein frozen specimens of tumor tissue taken from affected children in Uganda.[8]

For two years Epstein and his coworkers' attempts to isolate a virus using standard techniques and electron microscopy were unsuccessful. They then decided to grow Burkitt lymphoma cells in vitro, away from host defenses to allow the hypothesized oncogenic virus to replicate. Though previous attempts to establish cells of a lymphoid tumor in culture had failed, they were able to establish the first Burkitt lymphoma–derived cell line. Under the electron microscope, a cell in the first grid square showed particles that were recognizable as having a herpes virus morphology. Their results were published in the *Lancet* in 1964 in what has become a citation classic ("This Week's Citation Classic," Apr. 2, 1979).[9] The virus, which was named Epstein-Barr virus (EBV), was the first cancer-causing virus to be identified in humans. In the late 1970s the results of a large epidemiologic study in which blood samples were collected from forty-two thousand children between the ages of 4 and 8 years in the West Nile district of Uganda showed that children with high levels of antibodies to EBV, indicating past infection with the virus, were at high risk of developing Burkitt's lymphoma.[10] These findings strongly supported a causal relationship between EBV infection and the disease but suggested that the oncogenic potential of the virus is realized only in exceptional circumstances. Evidence later emerged that infection with malaria, which impaired resistance to the Epstein-Barr virus, was a necessary cofactor.[11]

Although Burkitt's lymphoma is the most common childhood cancer in areas where malaria is endemic (equatorial Africa, Brazil, and Papua New Guinea), it is extremely rare in other parts of the world, and the profound implications of the discovery of Epstein-Barr virus in Burkitt's lymphoma cells were not immediately apparent. Nevertheless, the work of Burkitt, Epstein, and colleagues spurred further research into the biological mechanism whereby the virus transformed lymphatic cells as well as the role of cofactors, such as malaria infection and immune status.[12] The Epstein-Barr virus is widespread, causing silent infections and infectious mononucleosis, and strikingly is associated with two human cancers, nasopharyngeal carcinoma as well as Burkitt's lymphoma.

* * *

During the precise years when Burkitt and his colleagues were documenting the extent of the occurrence of childhood lymphoma in equatorial Africa and developing chemotherapeutic treatments, a young German virologist, Harald zur Hausen, had completed his training and in 1966 had taken a postdoctoral position with the virologists Werner and Gertrude Henle at the Children's Hospital of Philadelphia. The Henles' laboratory was focused on the recently discovered Epstein-Barr virus. They had received EBV cell lines from Epstein's lab and were working to develop serologic markers of infection (that is, to detect antibodies to the virus in blood) for use in epidemiologic studies. In Philadelphia, zur Hausen requested to work on another virus (adenovirus) in order to familiarize himself with the techniques of molecular biology. To please his mentor, however, using the electron microscope, he demonstrated the presence of EBV particles directly in Burkitt's lymphoma cells that showed serologic evidence of infection, confirming the usefulness of the Henles' antibody test.

In 1969, having received an offer to set up his own research group at the University of Würzburg, zur Hausen returned to Germany and immediately decided to shift his focus entirely to EBV. His objective was to prove that EBV DNA persists in every tumor cell of Burkitt's lymphoma but does not establish a persistent infection there, as the Henles and others had assumed. In contrast to his mentors, who believed that only a minority of lymphoma cells harbored persistent infection, zur Hausen posited that EBV is present in all Burkitt's lymphoma cells and might be spontaneously reactivated. He obtained a large number of Burkitt's lymphoma cell lines and tumor biopsies, as well as material from nasopharyngeal carcinomas, which also appeared to be associated with EBV infection. Quickly overcoming the major obstacle, namely, the purification of adequate quantities of EBV DNA from a small number of virus-producing cells, he was able to show that a particular Burkitt's lymphoma cell line that was not actively producing EBV nevertheless contained multiple copies of EBV DNA in each cell. Soon after, using the new technique of in situ hybridization, zur Hausen was able to identify EBV genetic material in all Burkitt's lymphoma samples, as well as in samples of nasopharyngeal carcinoma, but not in any of the controls. He went on to demonstrate that the amount of viral material remained constant over time, suggesting an "intimate interaction of viral DNA with most, if not all, tumor cells." As he later wrote in his Nobel biography, "It seems that this was the first demonstration of persistent tumour virus DNA in human malignancies."[13]

During this period the Henles also demonstrated the causative role of the virus in infectious mononucleosis as well as the presence of EBV in nasopharyngeal carcinoma (the latter work involved zur Hausen). A summary of this work contained in the Henles' papers at the National Library of Medicine describes its significance as follows: "This significant relationship between Epstein-Barr virus and cancer demonstrated that the presence of certain viruses in the nucleus of a cell could transform a healthy cell into a malignant one."[14]

Zur Hausen was to maintain an interest in EBV and Burkitt's lymphoma throughout his career. In 1972, however, he was appointed chairman of the newly established Institute of Clinical Virology in Erlangen-Nürnberg. In his new position he decided to turn his attention to another cancer—cancer of the cervix—and a particular family of viruses—the papillomaviruses—which was to become the main focus of his energies. His work over the next eleven to twelve years was to radically transform our understanding of the role of viruses in human cancer, shedding light on this large and varied class of viruses, with momentous implications for the prevention and control of a major cancer in women worldwide, work that would eventually earn him a Nobel Prize.

The human papillomaviruses (HPVs) are small, double-stranded DNA viruses wrapped in a protein shell that have coexisted with the human species for hundreds of thousands of years, undergoing relatively few changes in their genetic makeup. Among the more than one hundred different HPV types that have been identified, some have an affinity for colonizing the skin, where they can produce warts, while others are adapted to the lining of the genital tract and other internal tissues. A third group is equally at home in either environment.[15]

Cervical cancer is a malignant neoplasm arising from the cells lining the cervix. Most cervical cancers are squamous cell carcinomas arising in the squamous, or flattened, epithelial cells lining the outer surface of the cervix. Adenocarcinoma arising in the glandular epithelial cells is the second most common type.

The earliest observations linking cervical cancer to a sexually transmitted agent date from the nineteenth century. In 1842 the Italian physician Domenico Antonio Rigoni-Stern had observed that cervical cancer rarely occurred in unmarried women and was virtually nonexistent among nuns, in contrast to its occurrence in married women, widows, and, particularly, prostitutes.[16] Later studies indicated that the disease was much rarer among women in certain religious groups, including Jews, the Amish, Mormons, and Seventh Day Adventists.[17] In the 1970s cervical cancer was the most common cancer occurring in women worldwide—today it is the fourth most common, surpassed only by cancers of the breast, intestines, and lung. Its highest rates were—and still are—seen in developing countries, particularly in East Africa, Central America, and the Pacific Islands.[18] Both internationally and within countries, cervical cancer incidence was associated with lower socioeconomic status. In the United States, cervical cancer rates are 45 percent higher among black women and 65 percent higher among Hispanic women compared to white women.[19]

Epidemiologic studies had identified a number of risk factors for cervical cancer in addition to socioeconomic status, including religion, having a larger number of children, use of oral contraceptives, smoking, and possibly nutrition. The two strongest and most consistent risk factors, however, were an early onset of sexual activity and a history of multiple sexual partners.[20] These findings pointed to an infectious agent as a cause of the disease, though by the end of the 1960s there was no solid evidence implicating a particular agent. Around this time the first reports appeared suggesting infection with Herpes simplex virus type 2 (HSV-2) as an agent in cervical cancer etiology, and HSV-2 became the prime suspect.[21] But over the next decade, attempts to isolate HSV-2 particles in cells from cervical cancers were uniformly unsuccessful, and large-scale epidemiologic studies failed to support a role of the virus. Zur Hausen, together with a coworker, had also failed in his efforts to find evidence of HSV-2 infection in cervical carcinoma.[22] This is where things stood when he returned to Germany.

In addition to the epidemiologic evidence implicating a transmissible agent in the development of cervical cancer, another body of work had contributed to zur Hausen's thinking. Looking back in a recent interview on how he came to focus on HPV and cervical cancer, he explained, "I was only interested in cervical cancer."[23] His attention had been directed to papillomaviruses by going back to the literature from the 1930s, when the researchers Richard Shope and Peyton Rous had observed lentil-like structures in wild U.S. cottontail rabbits. By taking cell-free extracts from these lesions and injecting them into domestic rabbits, they were able to produce similar warts that eventually became malignant. Zur Hausen had also come across anecdotal reports regarding genital warts that had occasionally converted gradually to malignant tumors. "These findings triggered the idea that there may be an agent in the genital lesions that could also cause cervical cancer."[24]

After the failure to find a link between HSV-2 and cervical cancer, in 1972 zur Hausen and his group started to work experimentally on HPV. He was convinced that genital warts were caused by a virus. He had observed HPV particles in genital warts and felt that HPV would be a "good candidate" for the infectious cause of cervical carcinoma.[25]  In 1973 at a meeting in Key Biscayne, Florida, he proposed that HPV was the cause of cervical cancer, but, given the prevailing consensus favoring HSV-2, his proposal met with little interest. Zur Hausen had collected a few hundred warts from individual patients and had isolated wart viruses from the skin of the hands and feet. But, to his disappointment, the wart virus could not be detected in cervical cancer biopsies or in genital warts. This was the first hint that there must be different types of human papillomavirus. Owing to the small number of viral particles in genital warts, it took zur Hausen and his colleagues several years to characterize and isolate HPV type 6 from a genital wart—this was achieved in 1977.[26] This type also could not be detected in carcinoma specimens. The researchers persisted, however, and a year later they found a related virus—HPV-11—in genital warts. Using HPV-11 as a probe and relaxing the stringency of the assay, they finally managed to isolate the distantly related HPV-16 and HPV-18 and, eleven years after embarking on this effort, to "link them convincingly to cancer." Reflecting, in an interview with the journal Nature (2012), on the painstaking path that led to the discovery, zur Hausen commented, "It was not a Eureka moment."[27]

As often happens with radically new ideas, the scientific community treated zur Hausen's findings dismissively. Infectious disease researchers, who had devoted years to investigating the role of HSV-2 and other sexually transmitted infections in cervical cancer, were unpersuaded; tumor virologists were skeptical in the absence of evidence demonstrating how the virus initiated cancer; and epidemiologists wanted to see data from carefully designed studies of human populations demonstrating a convincing association. While epidemiological and serologic studies had quickly linked hepatitis B virus with liver cancer, EBV with B-cell lymphomas, and Helicobacter pylori infections with gastric cancer, it took longer to work out and validate the serologic markers of HPV infection and to scale up the HPV molecular hybridization assays from the basic research laboratory to the clinical research laboratory to enable processing of the thousands of specimens needed in epidemiologic studies.[28]  It took nearly another decade of intensive research into the natural history of HPV infection and the epidemiology of cervical cancer before the cancer community accepted the evidence that HPV was the cause of the disease.

The bafflement regarding the causes of cervical cancer just before the identification of HPV-16 and HPV-18 is captured in a review article by Barbara Hulka, an epidemiologist at the University of North Carolina, summarizing the state of knowledge regarding the etiology of cervical cancer in the early 1980s:

> Despite a long history of research into the epidemiology and biology of cervical carcinoma, a definitive statement about its probable causes still remains elusive. . . . Although vigorously pursued, an increased risk from oral contraceptives has not been convincingly demonstrated. A variety of venereally transmitted organisms appear to be frequent cohabitants with cervical neoplastic cells. Herpesvirus type 2 still remains the prime suspect in the complex pathogenesis of cervical neoplasia. Clinical findings, biological characteristics of the virus, serological studies and interactions of host cells and viral particles continue to stimulate the most intensive investigative efforts.[29]

Only in the final paragraph did Hulka mention the link between genital warts and cervical dysplasia and HPV, stating, "A role of this virus in the development of cervical cancer has not yet been demonstrated." The next year zur Hausen would publish his definitive results implicating the high-risk HPV-16 as a cause of cervical cancer.[30]

A number of factors contributed to the difficulty of establishing that HPV played a causative role in cervical cancer. First, papillomaviruses are virtually ubiquitous on human skin and are widespread in the epithelial cells that form the lining of anogenital tissues, and it is difficult to determine whether evidence of viral infection in tumor cells points to causation or whether the virus is merely a "passenger" or "bystander," "cohabiting," as Hulka had put it, in cervical cancer cells.

Second, as research into HPV progressed, the number of specific types continued to grow, and at present well over one hundred types have been identified. Only a minority of HPV types are associated with cancer.[31]

Third, several features of the virus made it difficult to study. It is not easily cultured in the laboratory, and infected individuals do not mount a consistent antibody response, limiting the use of antibody levels in the blood for identifying viral types. This has meant that historically the only way to identify HPV has been from biopsies of warts or lesions. Further-more, the molecular techniques for detecting viral particles and for ampli-fying viral DNA in the 1970s and 1980s were cumbersome and insensitive. These were to undergo dramatic improvements with in situ hybridization and culminating in the development of polymerase chain reaction, or PCR, in 1983. PCR made it possible to amplify a single or a few copies of a piece of DNA by orders of magnitude, generating thousands to millions of copies of a particular DNA sequence.

A final factor that complicated the analysis and interpretation of the role of HPV infection in the cancer process was the lack of understand-ing of the "natural history" of cervical cancer, that is, the fact that cervical malignancy is the end result of a gradual progression from normal tissue to mild abnormalities to increasingly distorted behavior of the cells lining the cervix and finally to invasive cancer.[32] The process culminating in ma-lignancy typically unfolds over a period of fifteen to twenty years. Further obscuring the role of HPV in the carcinogenic process was the fact that, in most cases, early and even intermediate stages of dysplasia undergo spon-taneous regression to normal epithelium (referred to as "clearance" of the infection).[33] It took years of research examining the acquisition of HPV infections in young women and then following them over a period of years to appreciate that most HPV infections resolved on their own owing to the body's immune defenses, and that persistence of the virus leading to advanced dysplasia and ultimately to invasive cancer was relatively rare.[34] Robert Burk, pediatrician at the Albert Einstein College of Medicine, who got involved in studying HPV in the early 1980s, did early work that con-tributed to clarifying the natural history of the virus. He carried out one of the first studies showing that the prevalence of infection was strongly age-dependent—rates of infection were highest in young women and then declined, reflecting clearance of the virus.[35]

Until the natural history of the progression to cervical cancer was understood, there seemed to be a disconnect between the high incidence of HPV infections in the general population and the comparatively much lower incidence of invasive cervical cancer.[36]

* * *

HPV is the most common sexually transmitted infection worldwide. It in-fects roughly 10 percent of women at any given point in time, making it a "universal and pandemic" infection, as one researcher put it to me. Most women in the world will be infected by the virus at some point in their lives.[37] The highest rates of infection are seen in women in their teens and early twenties—those most sexually active—after which the rates decline with age, although there is a second lower peak around the age of menopause. In young women in the United States the prevalence of infection is about 25 percent.[38] These infections are, for the most part, transient and regress spontaneously. Ninety-five percent of lesions disappear within two years on their own and are of no clinical significance. However, in 5 to 10 percent of infected women, the infection persists and can result in precancerous lesions, which, if not removed, can progress to invasive cervical cancer. Thus cervical cancer is the end result of gradual progression of cellular pathology from normal tissue to increasingly abnormal features, and finally to invasive cancer.[39] The progression to invasive cancer normally takes decades, and this accounts for the success in the second half of the twentieth century in preventing cervical cancer in developed countries by widespread Papanicolaou (Pap) screening in which cells from the cervix are sampled and examined under a microscope. Regular Pap screening is effective because the cervix is accessible to clinical examination and because, once detected, precancerous lesions can be excised.

Of the more than one hundred HPV types, about fifteen are high-risk types for cervical cancer. Chief among these are, first and foremost, HPV-16 and, secondarily, HPV-18. The predominant role of HPV-16 is underscored by the fact that it is present in less than 3 percent of normal cervical tissues but is present in 20 percent of low-grade dysplasia, 45 percent of high-grade dysplasia, and 50 percent of invasive cancers. Together HPV-16 and 18 are responsible for roughly 70 percent of cervical cancer globally.[40]

Researchers at the National Cancer Institute recently summarized the significance of the natural history and the multistage process of HPV infection for the development of cervical cancer as follows: "The stages of cervical carcinogenesis include HPV infection; persistence, rather than clearance of the virus, linked to the development of a high-grade precursor lesion or 'precancer'; and invasion. *These are the necessary stages; cervical cancer is virtually impossible in the absence of sexually transmitted HPV infection and in the absence of intermediate progression to precancer*" (emphasis added).[41]

With the identification of specific HPV types associated with developing genital warts and cervical cancer, research into human papillomavirus and its role in cervical cancer intensified starting in the 1980s. The rate of acceleration is conveyed by the number of PubMed citations containing the terms "human papillomavirus" and "cervical cancer" over the past forty years: 1 in 1974, 5 in 1980, 81 in 1985, 221 in 1990, 432 in 2000, and 988 in 2010. Studies addressed different aspects of HPV infection with specific types and its role in cervical carcinogenesis. As the results of these studies appeared, they helped resolve poorly understood issues, fill in important gaps, and raise new questions. The HPV story is a powerful example of the painstaking, incremental progress between many groups working independently and collaboratively. Inevitably, there were missteps, misconceptions, and cumbersome and insensitive laboratory methods. But there was also a fortunate confluence of enormous energy, new insights, sharing of samples and results, and improved laboratory methods, which helped move the field forward.[42] Major results were replicated and extended, and concepts were refined and reformulated, contributing to filling out the picture of a major scientific and public health problem.

The identification of carcinogenic HPV genotypes in the mid-1980s spurred epidemiologists to undertake population-based studies to characterize the association of HPV infection with cervical cancer and precancer, and to determine whether HPV infection—the hypothesized cause—was consistent with the already identified risk factors, principally, age at first intercourse and number of lifetime sexual partners. The results of early epidemiologic studies were inconsistent, however, and suggested only a weak association of HPV exposure with disease. The uncertainty surrounding these studies reflected the facts that the definition of a precancerous lesion is somewhat subjective and that the different methods used to test for HPV seropositivity had variable sensitivity and accuracy.[43]

It took carefully designed studies carried out over more than a decade to improve the accuracy of these tests and establish reliable criteria for identifying women at high risk of developing cervical cancer. Researchers at the National Cancer Institute, led by Mark Schiffman, have been in the forefront of these efforts. As the criteria for defining high-risk cytology improved and the sensitivity of methods for detecting high-risk HPV DNA increased, the strength of the observed associations increased dramatically. The fact that this sharpening of measures of both exposure and disease outcome led to a strengthening of the association provided compelling support for a causal relationship.

Broadly speaking, three distinct types of studies contributed to elucidating major aspects of the HPV-cervical cancer relationship, and their results converged to provide overwhelming evidence that HPV was the obligatory cause of the disease. First, studies of the natural history of HPV infection, as described earlier, showed that persistent infection with high-risk types was necessary to cause cervical cancer. Second, large coordinated surveys documenting the prevalence of HPV infection with different HPV types in women with normal cytology were carried out in different countries throughout the world under the aegis of the International Agency for Research on Cancer.[44] These studies made it possible to compare the rates of infection in different regions with greatly differing socioeconomic conditions, health care systems, sexual mores, and rates of cervical cancer. Third, case-control and prospective studies conducted in different countries made it possible to gauge the magnitude of the association of HPV infection (any HPV infection, as well as infection with specific high-risk types) and the risk of cervical cancer. These studies took into account other risk factors for cervical cancer in addition to HPV infection, thereby enabling researchers to assess the relative importance of different risk factors. The results of these different types of studies complemented and buttressed one another and led to a three-dimensional and therefore much more convincing picture of the relationship of the virus to cervical cancer.

It was not until the early and mid-1990s that the results of large, population-based investigations and epidemiologic studies of HPV infection and cervical cancer began to appear. Under the auspices of IARC, an international survey of the prevalence of HPV infection among cervical cancer cases was carried out. Over a thousand frozen biopsy specimens were collected from twenty-two countries around the world. In each center, collaborators recruited fifty consecutive cases of invasive cervical cancer. A major strength of this study was that all specimens underwent centralized pathology review and centralized testing for HPV DNA in the tumor by PCR.[45] Initially, HPV DNA was detected in 93 percent of the specimens using PCR. However, when the 7 percent of specimens that initially tested negative were retested using a more sensitive technique, and when specimens were limited to those with clear evidence of malignancy, the prevalence of HPV DNA was 99.7 percent.[46] This provided strong evidence that HPV was a necessary cause of cervical cancer. In other words, in the absence of HPV infection there would be virtually no cervical cancer. As the McGill epidemiologist Eduardo Franco has pointed out, "This is the first instance in which a necessary cause has been demonstrated in cancer epidemiology."[47]

In the 1980s and 1990s epidemiologic studies—both case-control and prospective studies—were carried out in different countries to determine the magnitude of the risk of developing cervical cancer associated with HPV exposure. In addition to information on infection with HPV, studies typically gathered information on other exposures that might be independent risk factors or might modify the effect of HPV exposure. By the mid-1990s the results of these studies had demonstrated clearly and consistently that, after other factors were taken into account, HPV exposure (defined as the presence of HPV DNA in tumor specimens) was associated with a dramatically increased risk. In fact, the risk estimates from these studies are the highest found in epidemiologic studies of any cancer. A woman with evidence of infection with any HPV type has a relative risk of developing cervical cancer ranging from 50 to 100 (i.e., a fifty- to one hundred-fold increased risk). Women with evidence of infection with HPV-16 and HPV-18 have relative risks ranging from 100 to 500. And in some studies, the risk estimates reach values of between 500 and 1,000.[48] For comparison, compared to someone who has never smoked, a heavy smoker may have a twenty- to fiftyfold increased risk of developing lung cancer, depending on how many cigarettes he or she usually smoked per day.

Work in the early 1990s seemed to point to a mechanism by which HPV-16 initiates the carcinogenic process. HPV DNA becomes integrated into the host cell's genome—a process believed to be irreversible—leading to the inactivation of tumor suppressor genes and the immortalization of transformed cells.[49] Two critical viral proteins, known as E6 and E7, appear to interfere with cellular proteins involved in the regulation of the cell cycle, leading to uncontrolled cell growth and transformation to malignancy.[50]

The accumulation of scientific evidence from virology, molecular biology, and clinical and epidemiologic studies in many different countries provided strong support for a causal association of infection with specific HPV genotypes with risk of cervical cancer. This evidence can be summarized in terms of the "criteria for judging causal associations" discussed in chapter 2. As noted above, the association of HPV infection with risk of developing cervical cancer is the strongest in the field of cancer epidemiology. The association is consistent across studies carried out in different populations. There is a dose-response relationship between markers of persistent infection and risk (i.e., risk increases dramatically with markers of viral persistence). Prospective studies of young women demonstrate that infection with HPV precedes the development of disease by several decades. Epidemiologic evidence coheres with molecular pathologic evidence. Finally, evidence from molecular biology that HPV DNA is integrated into the host genome and is carcinogenic provides a mechanism, thereby satisfying the criterion of biological plausibility.[51]

The demonstration that persistent infection with HPV is the necessary cause of cervical cancer informs the interpretation of other potential risk factors, such as smoking, oral contraceptive use, number of live births, diet, and infection with other transmissible agents. The contribution of these other cofactors is modest compared to that of infection with a high-risk HPV type, as reflected in relative risks of between two- and threefold. As the sensitivity of assays for HPV increased, the relative risk estimates for these cofactors decreased; hence the elevated risk estimates may partially reflect residual confounding, since most of these variables are markers of sexual activity. Any role of these factors must now be understood in the context of their ability to modify (either enhancing or inhibiting) the process of HPV-initiated carcinogenesis. As researchers at the National Cancer Institute wrote, "Because HPV infection is a necessary cause of cervical cancer worldwide, no other risk factors are important in the absence of HPV, a somewhat startling conclusion that greatly affects usual epidemiologic approaches to effect modification and confounding."[52]

* * *

Although the cervix is the leading cancer site associated with HPV infection, the virus can also replicate and take hold in the cells that line the anogenital tissues generally and the throat of both sexes. Shortly after the identification of HPV-16 and 18 DNA in cervical cancer biopsies in 1983 and 1984, respectively, these HPV types, as well as several others, were found in other anogenital cancers.[53] Sites associated with HPV infection now include the vulva, vagina, penis, anus, and oropharynx. The proportion of cancer attributable to HPV is roughly 50 percent for vulvar cancer, 30–50 percent for penile cancers, and 60–90 percent for cancer of the vagina and anal and perianal cancers.[54] However, these cancers are extremely rare compared to cervical cancer.

A possible role of an infectious agent in the development of oropharyngeal cancer was suggested by a study in 1975 indicating that women with cervical cancer had a five- to sixfold increased risk of going on to develop oral cancer.[55] But it was not until 1985 that direct evidence established the presence of specific HPV types (principally HPV-16) in squamous cell carcinomas of the tongue and other subsites within the oropharynx. Between one-quarter and one-third of these cancers are now thought to be caused by anogenital high-risk HPV infections. In the past, most oropharyngeal cancers, like all head and neck cancers, had been strongly associated with two "traditional" risk factors, namely, smoking and heavy alcohol consumption. In spite of recent decreases in rates of other head and neck cancers, however, incidence rates of oropharyngeal cancer have increased dramatically since the 1980s, particularly in heterosexual, middle-aged men, mostly nonsmokers and nondrinkers. This change in the pattern of occurrence of oral cancer has been ascribed to changes in sexual behavior, including an increased number of sexual partners and an increase in oral-genital sexual practices predominantly among younger people starting in the 1970s.

Oropharyngeal cancers associated with HPV and those associated with smoking and drinking differ in a number of ways. HPV-associated oropharyngeal cancers tend to occur at the base of the tongue, in the tonsils, and in the back of the throat, whereas smoking- and alcohol-associated oral cancer has a wider distribution within the oral cavity. In addition, the prognosis of HPV-positive oropharyngeal cancer is much more favorable than that of the HPV-negative type—a difference that may partly be due to the absence of mutations in p53, a major tumor suppressor gene, which are a hallmark of the traditional oropharyngeal cancer. These differences, together with the contrasting profiles of those who develop the two types of oral cancer, have led researchers to conclude that HPV-negative and HPV-positive oral cancers represent two distinct diseases.[56]

Whereas the incidence of cervical cancer declined markedly in the United States from 1985 to 2005 and is expected to decline further by 2025, the incidence of oropharyngeal cancer has increased, and, strikingly, the proportion of these squamous cell carcinomas attributable to HPV infection has surged—from an estimated 16 percent in 1985 to an estimated 72 percent in 2005. And the proportion is projected to reach 90 percent by 2025.[57]

The role of HPV infection as a novel risk factor for oropharyngeal carcinoma received widespread media attention in July 2013, when the actor Michael Douglas announced that his throat cancer was caused by his having engaged in oral sex.[58] However, there is little public awareness of HPV infection as a risk factor for oral cancer. And, in contrast to the use of Pap testing for lesions of the cervix, no premalignant lesion has been identified for HPV-induced oropharyngeal cancer that could be used for screening.

Based on combining the number of cases at all anatomic sites, the total number of cancers that are associated with HPV infection in the United States in a given year is approximately thirty-one thousand.[59]

\* \* \*

In the first half of the twentieth century, cervical cancer was one of the most common cancers among women and a leading cause of cancer death among women in the United States. With the incorporation of Papanico-laou testing into gynecologic practice starting in the 1950s, cervical cancer mortality in the United States has declined by roughly 75 percent, and inci-dence has declined by half during the same period. The American Cancer Society estimated that there would be 12,900 new cases in 2015 and 4,100 deaths due to cervical cancer. Today cervical cancer now ranks fourteenth among female cancers in terms of incidence. Similar declines have taken place in other advanced industrial societies, and the widespread use of Pap testing has been credited with averting an epidemic of cervical cancer in the United Kingdom over the past several decades.[60]

Although Pap screening is credited with preventing many deaths from cervical cancer, it has serious limitations. Evaluation of Pap smears under the microscope is somewhat subjective, and it can miss precancerous le-sions. Follow-up and treatment of women with ambiguous cytology find-ings entails an enormous burden on the health care system and on women. Because Pap testing has a substantial false positive rate, many women un-dergo colposcopy (examination of the cervix with a magnifying device) and repeated testing when, in fact, their risk of developing cervical can-cer is low. The annual cost of these procedures has been estimated at four billion dollars. Finally, Pap testing cannot detect adenocarcinoma of the cervix, which for this reason has been increasing in incidence, while the more common squamous cell carcinoma has declined. Adenocarcinoma is caused principally by HPV-18.

In a landmark decision, in March 2014 an FDA panel unanimously rec-ommended that the Pap test be replaced with HPV-DNA testing. The new test detects HPV-16 and HPV-18, which account for 70 percent of cervical cancer cases. Testing for high-risk HPV DNA in cervical tissues represents an enormous advance in the ability to identify women who are truly at high risk and to reduce overtreatment of women at low risk. HPV DNA testing makes it possible to classify women very finely as to their risk. The test may reveal that one woman has a 60 percent chance of developing in situ cancer of the cervix within five years, whereas another woman has virtually no chance of developing cancer.[61]

An added benefit is that, owing to the greater accuracy of HPV DNA testing, women who test negative for high-risk types will be able to go with-out screening for three to five years. This is referred to as the test's "negative predictive value." According to Burk, "That's a really big deal. The nega-tive predictive value of a negative HPV DNA test is phenomenal." To Burk, who was a member of the FDA panel, the decision represents "a historic moment." "So you have the vaccine and you have the transformation of evidence-based medicine, where we really can now put into practice what we've learned about the epidemiology of HPV."[62]

* * *

By the early 1990s new insight into the natural history and epidemiology of HPV infection with specific high-risk genotypes opened up the possibility of developing a vaccine against HPV infection that would prevent cervical cancer. A highly effective vaccine against hepatitis B virus (HBV), a major cause of primary liver cancer in Asia and southern Africa, had been in use since the 1980s.

Soon after identifying HPV-16 and 18 in the mid-1980s, zur Hausen had tried to interest the pharmaceutical industry in the prospect of developing a vaccine against HPV infection. But his overtures met with little interest. Then, in the early 1990s, researchers in Australia and at the National Institutes of Health perfected the synthesis of empty virus-like particles (VLPs) from the HPV-16 protein shell, which triggers immunity to the virus.[63] Shortly thereafter, vaccine trials demonstrated that VLPs for species-specific papillomavirus prevented infections and tumors in cows, rabbits, and dogs. This work prompted pharmaceutical companies to pursue the technology to develop HPV vaccines.[64]

By 2006 the FDA had approved two vaccines for prevention of HPV infection. Merck's Gardasil is a quadrivalent vaccine, which targets HPV-16 and 18 as well as HPV-6 and 11, the most common types causing genital warts. Glaxo-Smith-Kline's Cervarix is a bivalent vaccine targeting HPV-16 and 18. Since it would take decades to determine whether the vaccines protected against cervical cancer, the FDA and other agencies decided to judge the efficacy of the vaccine based on how effective vaccination was in preventing precancerous cervical lesions. Both vaccines have been shown to be highly efficacious, conferring high levels of protection (greater than 90 percent) against persistent infection with HPV-16 and 18. Based on the studies carried out to date, this protection lasts undiminished for nearly a decade, and studies are currently in progress to assess protection afforded by the vaccines through at least fourteen years.[65] For the vaccine to be effective, it must be administered before the onset of sexual activity. For this reason, the Centers for Disease Control and Prevention (CDC) recommends that all girls be given either vaccine at 11 or 12 years of age and that boys be vaccinated with Gardasil at 11 or 12 years old. Both vaccines require three doses. So far, however, the response to the FDA recommendation has been disappointing. In spite of the vaccine's safety and efficacy, according to the CDC, as of 2014 only 40 percent of girls and only 22 percent of boys had received all three doses of the vaccine.[66] The much poorer compliance with HPV vaccination compared to other childhood vaccinations appears to be largely due to parents' and physicians' reluctance to confront the topic of sex, even though behavioral research demonstrates that teens who receive the HPV vaccine are no more likely to engage in casual or unsafe sex than those who do not.[67]

The most important outstanding question regarding HPV immunization is whether the vaccine will provide lifelong immunity or whether one or more booster shots will be required later in life. A second question is whether vaccination protects against infection at other sites, such as the oropharynx. In addition, for use in developing countries there is an urgent need for alternatives to the current vaccines, which are type-specific and expensive and require cold chain transportation.

Since HPV-16 and 18 infections account for approximately 70 percent of all cervical cancers, second-generation vaccines are being developed that would cover over 90 percent of the cancer-causing HPV genotypes, including, in addition to HPV-16 and 18, HPV-45, 31, 33, 52, 35, 58, 39 (highly prevalent in Latin America), and 51 (highly prevalent in Africa). The results of a clinical trial comparing a new "nonavalent" vaccine (i.e., targeting nine different HPV types) to the quadrivalent vaccine have demonstrated protection against five additional HPV types.[68]

\* \* \*

Although its incidence has been dramatically reduced in developed countries due to Pap testing, cervical cancer is the third most common cancer among women worldwide and causes the largest number of cancer-related deaths among women in developing countries. According to estimates from IARC's GLOBOCAN program, each year there are 530,000 new cases of cervical cancer worldwide and 275,000 deaths from the disease.[69] The vast majority of the burden of cervical cancer—more than 85 percent of new cases and 88 percent of deaths—occurs in the developing world, giving it the most inequitable burden of any cancer. Without changes in prevention and control, due solely to population growth and aging of the population, cervical cancer deaths are projected to reach 430,000 annually by 2030, virtually all in developing countries.

Mortality from cervical cancer varies widely internationally (fig. 7.2). Age-standardized mortality rates are highest in East and West Africa,

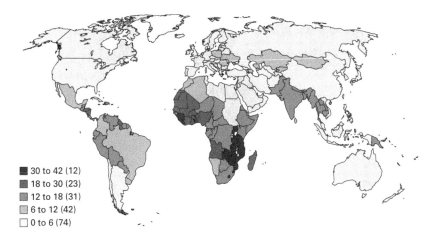

30 to 42 (12)
18 to 30 (23)
12 to 18 (31)
6 to 12 (42)
0 to 6 (74)

Figure 7.2
Geographic distribution of age-standardized cervical cancer mortality by country. The counts in parentheses in the legend correspond to the number of countries in each mortality rate range.
Adapted from Arbyn et al. 2011. By permission of Oxford University Press.

intermediate in Southern Africa, South-Central Asia, South America, and Central Africa, and lowest in West Asia, North America, and Australia/New Zealand. There is a tenfold difference between the rates in the highest versus the lowest mortality regions of the world. Although the highest rates are seen in East Africa, it is India, with an intermediate mortality rate and a population of 1.3 billion, that had the largest number of deaths from cervical cancer (72,824) and accounts for roughly a quarter of the worldwide burden of cervical cancer.[70] The death rate from cervical cancer in less developed countries is on average roughly three times that in more developed countries. In the developing world cervical cancer kills women in their prime who are often the sole support of young children. Thus it exacts an enormous toll in terms of premature death, years of life lost, and family and societal impacts.[71]

The substantial variation in cervical cancer rates largely reflects the pattern of screening availability in different parts of the world. The low mortality areas of the map in figure 7.2 are those in which Pap screening is available. If one had drawn such a map a century ago, before the introduction of Pap testing, mortality rates from cervical cancer would be much more uniform throughout the world, reflecting the universal distribution of HPV.

The global prevalence of HPV infection in the cervix in women with normal cytology at any given point in time is about 10 percent. As shown

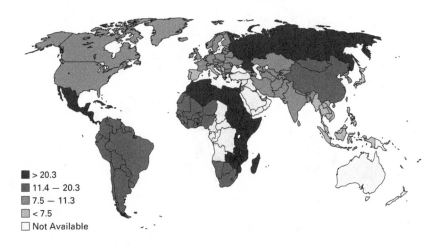

Figure 7.3
Estimated HPV DNA prevalence in different regions of the world. Estimates are based on a meta-analysis of 78 studies, including 157,879 women with normal cytology. Shading represents the adjusted prevalence in the region and denotes the quartile distribution of all the estimates.
*Source*: Sanjosé et al. 2007. By permission of Elsevier.

in figure 7.3, HPV prevalence does vary by region, although not as much as incidence or, especially, mortality from cervical cancer. Rates are generally higher in low-income countries compared to those in more developed regions. Women in Africa, and in particular in East Africa, have the highest HPV prevalence rates (32 percent), while the lowest estimates are seen in Southeast Asia (6 percent). These differences in the prevalence of HPV infection in the general population likely reflect cultural norms affecting sexual behavior, such as age at first marriage, marriage to older men or to men who have several contemporaneous partners, and poor hygiene.[72]

The recognition that infection with high-risk HPV types is the necessary cause of virtually all cervical cancers has created an unprecedented opportunity—and implicitly, an ethical obligation—with regard to a major cause of cancer deaths in the developing world. That is to say, through a combination of screening and vaccination, there is the potential to drastically reduce the number of deaths from this disease. With the exception of liver cancer, this cannot be said of any other major cancer, such as those of the breast, colon, lung, prostate, endometrium, ovary, or leukemia or lymphoma.

\* \* \*

As a result of painstaking work over the past thirty years, the strategies and tools available for reducing morbidity and mortality from cervical cancer have been radically transformed.[73] Depending on the target age-group, one of two strategies is available. These are referred to as "primary prevention" and "secondary prevention." *Primary prevention* refers to preventing infection with high-risk HPV genotypes in preteens—before exposure to the virus. In theory, currently available prophylactic vaccines could prevent approximately 70 percent of cervical cancer in the future in girls vaccinated before the age of 12. *Secondary prevention* refers to screening of women who are already sexually active to identify and surgically remove precancerous lesions or cancers before they become life-threatening. Novel methods, referred to as "screen and treat," have been developed for use in low-resource countries with limited health care infrastructure. However, implementing these strategies in the places where they are most needed—in developing countries like Uganda and India—is anything but simple, and realizing the promise of HPV prevention research will require overcoming formidable obstacles.

These obstacles pervade all sectors of low-income societies, from the level of the household to that of government policy and international aid. The most immediate problems are a lack of health services and qualified staff, but at another level endemic corruption, government bureaucracy, and weak rule of law stand in the way of adopting the needed programs.[74] Furthermore, while preventing deaths from cervical cancer is an urgent need, developing countries face many other urgent needs competing for attention and scarce resources, including malnutrition, high infant mortality and maternal childbirth deaths, and lack of clean water and basic sanitation. At the same time, the incidence of chronic diseases, such as cancer, diabetes, and cardiovascular disease, is increasing owing to changes in society and lifestyle, principally, increasing tobacco use and obesity. Moreover, in some countries a disease that affects women only may not command as much support as other health problems. Beyond the question of material resources, attitudes toward vaccination can pose a serious obstacle in regions where there is mistrust among groups that may view government efforts to vaccinate young girls as part of a birth control program or, worse, as attempts to spread AIDS.[75]

In spite of these considerable obstacles, international agencies, nongovernmental organizations, pharmaceutical companies, donors, and ministries of health are working together to address the prevention of cervical cancer. A variety of demonstration projects are underway in developing countries to determine the most effective way to deliver the vaccine to pre-adolescent girls. In 2012 Uganda's Ministry of Health, in collaboration with Merck, Sharpe, and Dohm, launched a program to vaccinate 140,000 girls aged 9–12 with Gardasil. The program included twelve out of one hundred districts in the country. The GAVI Alliance, a public-private partnership including international agencies, pharmaceutical companies, donors, and governments, is supporting the introduction of HPV vaccination demonstration programs targeting 180,000 girls in eight developing countries, mainly in sub-Saharan Africa. These programs will provide valuable experience and preliminary data for the design of effective national vaccination programs. By 2015 GAVI planned to extend its pilot projects to reach approximately one million girls in twenty countries; and by 2020 the goal is to have vaccinated more than thirty million girls in over forty countries. In countries where the average per capita income is less than two dollars a day, cost is a serious issue, and GAVI is making the vaccine available in poor countries for $4.50 per dose.[76]

If these programs deliver on their promise, they will succeed in reaching and vaccinating preteen girls and will then be expanded to cover the entire populations of these countries. But sustained funding will be needed to support vaccination beyond the first wave as a permanent component of health care services. Once primary prevention through vaccination is assured, there will still be a vital need for screening programs for the female population above the age of thirteen who are still at risk of developing cervical cancer. Screening will also be essential to monitor the effectiveness of the vaccine as well as to detect cancers caused by types other than HPV-16 and HPV-18, which are included in currently available vaccines.[77]

One observer summed up what is at stake in developing countries as follows: "With the availability of an effective, safe vaccine, there is real hope for reducing the global burden of cervical cancer. Although achieving broad coverage of young adolescents, negotiated tiered pricing, and securing financing will be challenging, it is sobering to realize that with every 5-year delay in bringing vaccination to developing countries, 1.5 million to 2 million more women will die."[78]

Given what has been learned in the past thirty years, we are in the unprecedented situation of having the ability to virtually eradicate this type of cancer. All that stands in the way are practical issues of resources and strategies and the political leadership to realize the potential solution. This would be the first time in history that a type of cancer was eradicated. In speaking of the potential for eradicating cervical cancer, Burk pointed to the global eradication of smallpox in 1977, which was the culmination of a campaign by the World Health Organization, and lamented the lack of drive and energy to implement the required program. "We have the means to eliminate cervical cancer, if we had the energy that he had [D.A. Henderson—who led the smallpox eradication campaign]. Of course, smallpox is a different kind of disease—it is more immediate—but still, we have the means to do that now."[79]

The fact that HPV types have changed little over the past 200,000 years suggests that cervical cancer has been around at least since *Homo sapiens* diverged from other hominids. Yet only in the past thirty years has HPV been demonstrated to cause cancer in humans. The finding that infection with high-risk HPV types is estimated to cause 5 percent of all cancers worldwide underscores the momentousness of the present juncture.

* * *

If the HPV story ended here, it would qualify as one of the great achievements in cancer research, epidemiology, and global public health. But there is more to the story. The effort to identify high-risk carcinogenic HPV types and to understand how they induce cancer has led to a comprehensive cataloguing of the genetic differences both between and within viral types at a minute level. And an appreciation of the tremendous genetic variation within the Papillomaviradae family is yielding insights in several disparate fields. First, as the number of HPV types has grown, there is an increasing appreciation for the high degree of specialization and adaptation of the virus to its animal and human hosts. Second, a key question is why a minority of forms of the virus but not others are highly carcinogenic. Answering this question will contribute to understanding the carcinogenic process. Finally, comparison of HPV types and variants from cervical smears from different populations throughout the world has shown potential to shed new light on human evolution and human migrations.

Since zur Hausen isolated the first HPV types in the 1980s, the number of HPV types has steadily grown. At present 170 human and 20 animal papillomavirus genotypes have been fully characterized, and it is expected that more human and, particularly, animal genotypes will be identified in the future. Zur Hausen's wife Ethel-Michelle de Villiers maintains a reference center in Heidelberg, Germany, for the confirmation and cataloguing of new HPV types. A distinct genotype, or species, of papillomavirus is one that differs from other identified types by more than 10 percent in a key segment of the HPV genome. Each of the more than one hundred distinct types has been isolated either from abnormal growths in different tissues (skin, epithelial tissues of the cervix, vagina, vulva, anus, penis, or the oropharynx), including warts, precancer, or invasive cancer, or from normal tissues.

De Villiers has constructed a phylogenetic tree depicting known HPV types in terms of the degree of relatedness of different genotypes (fig. 7.4). The different types fall into three major groupings, or "genera," denoted by Greek letters alpha, beta, and gamma. The alpha types tend to colonize the

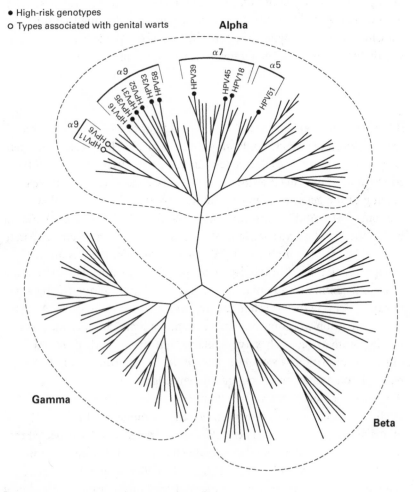

Figure 7.4
Phylogenetic tree showing 170 HPV types.
Adapted from De Villiers 2013. By permission of Elsevier.

mucous membranes, whereas the beta and gamma types are adapted more to the skin. All the types found today, which are denoted by the extremities of the branches, evolved from a common ancestor that existed hundreds of millions of years ago. Unlike the family trees in which time is represented along the horizontal or vertical axis, here as we move inward toward the center, where the "trunks" of the three major genera meet, we are moving back in time. The presumed common ancestor of all HPV types is located in the center of the diagram.

Looking at another phylogenetic tree, this one limited to HPV types in the alpha papillomavirus genus—which includes HPV-16—Burk stressed that the key thing is that every one of the types that causes cancer has a common origin. However, not all the viruses that have evolved from this common ancestor cause cancer. This suggests that the ability to adapt to an ecologic niche that causes cancer has been lost in some of the types. For example, the alpha 6 grouping, which is associated with genital warts, represents a completely different ecological niche from the alpha 9 and 7 groupings, which cause cancer. And other groupings are more or less benign. Most alpha HPV types coexist with the host and don't cause any pathology.

Burk told me that his real interest is in understanding the genetic basis of cervical cancer:

> The key observation is that HPV causes cervical cancer as collateral damage, not as part of its natural life cycle. In fact, it's the ones that cause cancer that have evolved into a certain ecological niche, where their survival is a little better and, unfortunately, there's an overlap between those traits and the dysregulation of a particular cell population—that is, cells of the squamo-columnar junction of the female cervix. The female has these specific cells at the squamo-columnar junction that the virus has adapted to—only certain HPV types—and, unfortunately, as part of their evolution and adaptation, they also cause cervical cancer.[80]

Differences in the genetic sequence of HPV types are believed to determine two independent traits, which are necessary for the virus to cause cancer—the ability to persist (i.e., to maintain infection) and to progress on the path to cancer. According to Burk, something about HPV-16 makes it "uniquely likely both to persist and to cause neoplastic progression when it persisted, making it a remarkably powerful human carcinogen." Other carcinogenic types, many related to HPV-16, were not particularly persistent but could cause neoplastic progression, at lower rates than HPV-16 if they did persist.

The "remarkable" pattern of differences in natural history between the types is prompting more detailed investigations, whose goal is to figure out what genetic variant—what specific piece of the HPV genome—makes it so carcinogenic. What is the difference between HPV-16 and its closest sister types, HPV-31 and HPV-35, that accounts for the former's much greater carcinogenic potential? Understanding this would provide an unprecedented insight into the mechanism of HPV carcinogenesis.

Using "whole genome sequencing," researchers are now in a position to examine the entire HPV genome, which is small enough to permit a comprehensive analysis of all its components and functions on a population level. This is the goal of a project that Burk and his colleagues have called the HPV Human Genome Project, which includes researchers at Einstein, the National Cancer Institute, IARC, and BGI, a high-powered genome sequencing company in Shenzhen, China. This approach has the potential to reveal genetic differences in the papillomavirus that, depending on its interaction with its human host, can have very large effects. For example, the different variant lineages of HPV-16 have associations with risk of cervical cancer on the order of sixfold. However, comparing HPV-16 to related types in the alpha-9 species group yields huge differences—perhaps fiftyfold. Given this powerful phenotypic difference (that is, whether one develops cervical precancer or cancer or not, depending on the viral genome), these new genome-phenotype correlation studies have a much better chance of yielding results than the human genomics studies have.

As Burk put it:

> The key to understanding the molecular basis of HPV carcinogenicity is realizing that the biological driving force has been the evolution of specific HPV's into discrete host ecosystems, such as the epithelium from the cervix, vagina, external genital skin, or skin covering other anatomic surfaces. Each bodily ecosystem has characteristics that allow adapted HPVs some type of competitive advantage to infect, replicate, and transmit. Nevertheless . . . HPV-16 stands out as having the most pathogenic phenotype (e.g., HPV-16 causes both cervix and oropharyngeal cancer).[81]

\* \* \*

The concerted effort to understand the human papillomavirus has been motivated by the virus's ability to induce cancer. But, as an unanticipated by-product of medically motivated research, studies of the variation in the virus have yielded insights in a totally different area. Because the papillomavirus phylogenetic tree includes genomes isolated from cervical smears from all over the world, this molecular variation simultaneously reflects geographic variation and differences in population groups.

The existence of stored samples of cervical smears from populations around the world has enabled researchers to use fine variation in the HPV genome as a means of reconstructing prehistoric viral spread and the movement of ancient populations. This is possible due to the tremendous diversity of HPV types and the fact that HPV variants show the greatest divergence when they are obtained from ethnic groups that evolved for a long time without contact, such as Africans and American Indians.[82] The finer (and more recent) variation within types and the greater variation distinguishing types can be used as an evolutionary clock to trace HPV speciation going back millions of years.

Using this logic, Hans-Ulrich Bernard and colleagues at the University of California at Irvine examined worldwide variation within HPV-18 in samples obtained from population groups in different parts of the world. They concluded that diversity within the HPV-18 genome correlates with patterns of evolution and the spread of *Homo sapiens* out of Africa. HPV-18 variants from Amazonian Indians were most closely related to those from Japanese and Chinese patients, in conformity with the posited dating of the migration of Asian peoples across the Bering Strait and down into the Americas approximately twelve thousand years ago. Bernard and colleagues speculated that the split between two closely related genotypes HPV-18 and HPV-45 occurred more than half a million years ago, and that speciation events between less closely related viral genotypes may have occurred "several million years ago, i.e., before the evolution of humans."[83]

Bernard and colleagues have carried out similar studies of HPV-16. The strongest pattern among HPV-16 variants pointed to the independent evolution of the virus among Africans, Caucasians, and East Asians and reflected colonization of the Americas by Europeans and Africans. As in the analysis of HPV-18, HPV-16 appears to have evolved over more than 200,000 years from a precursor genome that may have originated in Africa. The authors concluded that "the identification of molecular variants is a powerful epidemiological and phylogenetic tool for revealing the ancient spread of papillomaviruses, whose trace through the world has not yet been completely lost."[84]

The prevalence of different HPV types and variants within types in different populations worldwide reflects the history of the virus-host relationship at the most intimate level, which, in turn, is the outcome of in-numerable interactions over time between different groups, including con-quest, intermarriage, and migration. For genital HPVs, the fundamental interaction is the sexual encounter between groups carrying different HPV types. In the stark picture painted by Burk, the fundamental interaction comes down to an essential feature of human behavior:

> If you imagine the history of man, people are nasty, they go around and rape one group, and if the virus is eliminated before they found the next person, it would be gone—there would be no more papil-lomavirus. In another instance, one tribe will go and rape all the women in another tribe and just kill everybody, so their victims' genes wouldn't be perpetuated, but their HPV would be! So those types that we see today have persisted over time and allowed replication. Be-cause it's evolution—whatever replicates wins.[85]

It turns out that the project of mapping the genome of the virus and understanding its genetic variation is inextricably intertwined with under-standing the geographic distribution of different HPV types and variants and their evolution in tandem with the migrations of human and hominid populations, as well as the distribution of associated disease.

* * *

Looking back over the past three decades, in 2009 Burk summarized the fortunate "confluence" of a number of different factors that made possible the tremendous progress in the field encompassing basic research on HPV and its clinical implications. First, advances in technology (recombinant DNA, cloning of HPV genomes, and the use of molecular hybridization) represented a quantum advance over the standard virologic methods (i.e., serology), and these new methods were used in epidemiologic studies of disease. Second, the free and widespread distribution of cloned HPV ge-nomes by the Heidelberg group and the inauguration of an annual inter-national papillomavirus conference "fostered a collaborative culture within the PV community." "From a public health viewpoint, HPV has become the model for molecular medicine and how technology can be readily applied to global health problems."[86]

Others in the field of cancer epidemiology have argued that the HPV story provides a model for how basic science findings can be applied to

real-world problems and make an enormous difference in reducing morbidity and mortality. Rather than a narrow focus on etiology, epidemiologists are encouraged to adopt a broader ecologic model of population
health and to tackle issues of health care and survivorship.[87]

\* \* \*

The enormous distance traversed and the astonishing progress over the
past fifty years in understanding the role of viruses in the development of
cancer and in the prevention and control of fatal cancers is highlighted by
a story from Burkitt's later life. In 1964 Burkitt resigned his post at Mulago
Hospital in Kampala and two years later returned to England to work for
the Medical Research Council in London. After having spent eighteen years
in Uganda, he was left "at sea" by the move back to England and the lack of
clinical involvement with patients, and he had no idea whether he would
find any sort of occupation. As happened in his early career, however, another totally unanticipated opportunity was placed in his path. The eminent epidemiologist Sir Richard Doll introduced him to Peter Cleave, and
he was galvanized by Cleave's idea that many of the diseases of Western civ-
ilization could be ascribed to diet, and specifically to a high consumption of
refined carbohydrates and a lack of dietary fiber.[88] This new interest was to
preoccupy him for the rest of his life. In 1968, when Clifford Nelson, one of
his two companions on the tumor safari, visited him and asked him about
the latest on Burkitt's lymphoma, he replied, "Cliff, it's all out of my hands
now. All the really clever chaps in epidemiology, virology, immunology,
and biochemistry have left me in the dust."[89] This was only ten years after
the publication of his initial paper on Burkitt's lymphoma. Burkitt died in
1993. One can only guess what he would have made of the decades of research on HPV—with its impressive advances—that, in an important way,
grew out of his groundbreaking work on childhood lymphoma in Africa.

# Conclusion

In a pithy little book published in 2014 titled *Are We All Scientific Experts Now?*, the sociologist of science Harry Collins explored public attitudes toward science in an attempt to explain recent phenomena like the antivaccine movement and climate skepticism.[1] Collins noted that the public's trust in science has declined from its apogee in the decades following World War II, and he attributed this decline to a simplistic reading of Thomas Kuhn and the rise of social relativism, starting in the 1970s. He went on to provide a useful inventory of different types of expertise to distinguish what is special about *scientific* expertise. Collins's aim was to explain what it is about scientific activity that sets it apart from other activities we are familiar with, in order to restore science to the position it deserves. He held up as the epitome of real science physicists working on gravitation waves, who delayed publishing important results because their confidence in their measurements was not absolute.

However, both the circumstances and the culture of science in the area of biomedicine and public health differ in important respects from those of experimental physics. Physicists are not in the habit of lobbying the public to gain support for their particular point of view, and they are not given to claiming that their findings are politically correct. Furthermore, the public is not clamoring for answers to the mysteries of black holes and dark matter. Because the problems physicists study are so far removed from everyday life, they are able to pursue their work in relative isolation from external influences.

When it comes to the study of factors that may affect our health, the situation is quite different. Because research in this area focuses on clinical diseases affecting real people, the results appear to have a direct relevance to our lives. We are all eager for solid information that would permit us and our loved ones to avoid, or survive, the chronic diseases that are the major causes of death and disease in advanced societies. For this reason, findings from studies of disease have a particular power and mystique, which can influence what results are reported, how they are reported, and what is made of them in the wider society.

If research in public health were conducted out of the spotlight, one could leave it to internal mechanisms of the discipline and to time to weed out what stands up and what is important. But, as we have seen, the landscape in which health risks are studied and in which findings are disseminated is pervaded by false claims, oversold results, biases operating at the level of observational studies as well as psychological and cognitive biases, and professional and political agendas. On certain topics, as we have seen, scientists holding conflicting views cannot find common ground and are polarized into opposed camps, or "silos." Needless to say, this type of behavior is not in line with scientists' view of their profession nor with Collins's view of science.

If scientists disagree on many questions regarding health, nutrition, biotechnology, and the environment, it is small wonder that nonscientists are confused about what are arcane and difficult issues that require special expertise to begin to understand, no less to assess critically. Such questions—and the research that addresses them—only become more confused when they are catapulted into the public arena. Rather than being assessed on strictly scientific grounds, they are refracted through many different lenses according to the outlook or agenda of different groups or individuals. In many cases the resulting versions of the relevant science involve serious simplifications or distortions. Often the goal is to distill the results of a particular study, or of the totality of evidence on a question, to a simple yes/no dichotomy that either confirms or contradicts what we would like to believe. But there is no reason for us to expect that all studies on a difficult question will deliver a clear-cut answer, and much less that they will all line up "on the right side." Furthermore, as we have seen, all studies are not equal.

When difficult scientific questions are drastically simplified to fit a specific purpose or agenda—journalistic, regulatory, ideological, political, or personal—often the most basic distinctions and considerations are lost sight of. The mental fog produced by so much misinformation and partisan spinning of the science can be dispelled only by keeping in view certain fundamental facts that rarely get attention. These are worth reprising below.

There are real problems and there are false problems, that is, problems that, to the best of our knowledge, are not problems at all. Vaccines, genetically modified crops and foods, and cell phones are not threats to our well-being. Rather, they are among the greatest advances contributing to human welfare. We need to get better at distinguishing false problems from real problems.

Biology is complex, and we should not underestimate the difficulty of the problems we want to see solved. This difficulty helps explain why progress in understanding diseases such as pancreatic cancer, Alzheimer's, and many others' has been so slow. It also explains how dramatic advances can be made on some fronts, but, in spite of concerted efforts, progress on other fronts can be disappointing. Often we recite the meager knowledge we have on a question and fail to acknowledge just how little we actually know. Being open about our ignorance would both serve as an incentive to fill in the knowledge void and, at the same time, serve to highlight the real progress that has been made in answering other questions.

The quality of research and the rate of progress in uncovering new knowledge vary dramatically between different areas. For example, in the area of genetics and genomics there has been impressive progress, and high standards have been established for the replication of findings, allowing the field to move forward. In contrast, findings concerning environmental exposures and their effects on health are much weaker and are subject to controversy.[2] The fact is that there are fields where the methods and the hypotheses are more robust than those in other fields.

As we have seen, it is now widely recognized that much of what is published is either wrong or exaggerated and that there is an epidemic of false claims that gain wide circulation and are not easily dispelled, even when more solid contradictory evidence becomes available. False claims are fueled and reinforced by the many biases that affect both the scientific work and how it gets presented to the public. The true extent of false claims and misinformation in biomedicine has only recently begun to receive systematic study. The prevalence of error in the published literature points up the difficulty of the problems studied and the need for improved standards in research. It turns out that a lot of what we think we know is wrong.

How one approaches a question can have a decisive effect on how productive one's efforts will be. If one frames the issue in a way that screens out relevant considerations, it stands to reason that one is reducing one's chances of finding something new and important. This is the lesson that Richard Sharpe drew from twenty years of high-profile but fruitless efforts to find evidence supporting the endocrine disruption hypothesis. Rather than asking how exposure to endocrine disrupting chemicals in the environment causes reproductive disorders, he posed the question, what causes these disorders? As he commented, "Such a simple difference, but it takes your thought processes in a very different direction." We should note that Sharpe's restatement of the problem meant going against the tide, since it meant rejecting a fashionable idea that had wide support from the public and that improved one's chances of obtaining funding.

Sharpe also stresses that "getting it wrong is alright" and that failure is an essential part of the research process—that is, if it prompts one to take a fresh look at one's framing of the problem rather than cling to one's hypothesis.[3] Failure is an essential part of the research process because it forces one to go back and ask where one went wrong. If the work was done right, being led to a dead-end forces one to redirect one's attention to another, possibly more promising question.

In addition to framing the question in such a way as to maximize the possibility of finding a meaningful answer, there are other "simple" distinctions that can increase the chances of identifying a fruitful path. First and foremost is a consideration of the characteristics of the agent one is interested in. If the focus is "endocrine disrupting chemicals," one has to start by documenting the relative dose and potency of human exposures in different environments to these chemicals, which are hypothesized to be having detectable effects on the population. Since all researchers agree that the DES experience of pregnant women in the middle of the last century provides the cornerstone for studies of environmental estrogens, one would expect researchers to acknowledge the enormous difference in dose and potency between DES administered as a drug to these women and typical exposure to trace amounts of chemicals in the environment. However, this is rarely done. To recognize that the environmental exposure is many orders of magnitude weaker than the pharmacologic doses does not rule out that the former is worthy of study, but it does mean that any effects are likely to be much harder to detect, and also that research would not incite the kind of fear and certainty that it tends to in the public.

By our nature, we are disposed to want to find external causes to account for diseases we don't understand. These are things that are beyond our control, and this helps explain the enormous appetite for stories about what are extremely low-level exposures in the environment. Such low-level exposures may be having real effects and may well merit study. But we should keep in mind that the major causes of chronic disease that have been identified in the past sixty or so years are smoking, heavy alcohol consumption, heavy sun exposure, excess body weight, a poor diet, lack of physical activity, exposure to certain micro-organisms, and socioeconomic inequality. These are factors that have large effects. There are few things that are studied in the realm of public health that influence one's risk of disease by a factor of five, or ten, or more, but these factors do just that. And yet, curiously, these factors, which are mundane and appear to be under our control, do not inspire anywhere near the kind of fear that is inspired by trace exposures to "chemicals" and "radiation" in the environment.

As regards the future, we hear a great deal about the many exciting developments that have the potential to yield undreamed of advances— "precision medicine," "targeted therapies," "gene therapy," "regenerative medicine," "tissue engineering," and the use of "Big Data" to uncover new relationships in unprecedentedly rich datasets. Here too, however, we need to keep in mind how difficult and slow real progress on these fronts is likely to be and that, while these approaches may revolutionize the treatment of specific illnesses, they are less likely to transform our lives. Big Data, or "data mining," represents a powerful tool that can supplement or, in some cases, replace hypothesis-driven research, as in the search for genes linked to disease. As has been pointed out, however, the use of Big Data to solve meaningful problems will require much better data than are currently available, as well as new methods to analyze the data and to avoid spurious findings.[4] Although the project of understanding the role of genetics in complex diseases is certain to lead to fundamental change in how we prevent and treat disease, it is significant that Eric Lander, the head of the federal Human Genome Project, has cautioned that the real payoff from this work is generations away.

* * *

The exciting and beautiful thing is that an astute observation and the determination to solve a mystery can, in fortunate circumstances, lead to the formulation of a hypothesis that can transform our understanding of a problem and lead to new strategies to prevent or cure disease. This is what happened when Denis Burkitt, observing the swollen jaws of Ugandan children with a mysterious disease, thought to undertake a continent-wide survey that led to the first linkage between a virus and a human cancer. This is what happened when a Belgian pathologist noted the similarity between the type of kidney damage observed in women on a weight-loss regimen, which included Chinese herbs, in a Brussels clinic in the 1990s and that seen in patients with Balkan nephropathy. This is what happened when Arthur Grollman decided to undertake molecular studies of upper uro-thelial cancer in the Balkans and in East Asia—studies that demonstrated a unique type of genetic damage to the urinary tract caused by exposure to aristolochic acid. And this is what happened when Harald zur Hausen questioned the dogma that herpes simplex virus must be the cause of cer-vical cancer and made a connection between the observation of virus-in-duced lesions in cottontail rabbits in the 1930s and the pathology of human cervical cancer.

Much promising work is going on that will undoubtedly lead to new breakthroughs, although we cannot say where these will occur. When a breakthrough does come about, it is more likely to come from the persis-tent work of different groups pursuing a strong hypothesis that has been refined as a result of challenges and self-criticism than as a result of focus-ing on a culprit that appeals to our ill-defined fears and ignoring contradic-tory evidence and competing hypotheses. We need to promote a model of what science is and how it operates at its best, based on examples like those presented in the preceding chapters and described by many others. The achievements that we are surrounded by and that we often take for granted, for the most part, did not come about as the result of one individual's stroke of insight and certainly didn't come from following some fashionable but ill-defined idea. Rather they are the result of trying to answer an important question by building on and extending existing knowledge. Such achieve-ments required persistence and collaborative work conducted out of the spotlight by many different groups, each contributing a piece to the larger puzzle, with no guarantee that the work would turn out to be important. It is these real accomplishments that should serve as models of what science can achieve and, at the same time, provide a standard for judging over-stated claims, implausible findings, and appeals to irrational fear.

# Appendix
## *List of Interviews*

Robert K. Adair, professor emeritus, Physics Department, Yale University, New Haven, Conn.; in-person interview July 11, 2009; e-mail and telephone conversations.

Robert D. Burk, professor, Departments of Pediatrics; Microbiology and Immunology; Obstetrics & Gynecology and Women's Health; and Epidemiology and Population Health, Albert Einstein College of Medicine, Bronx, N.Y., March 25, 2014.

Daniel R. Doerge, research chemist, National Center for Toxicological Research, U.S. Food & Drug Administration, Jefferson, Ark.; e-mail interview January 2, 2015, and multiple e-mail exchanges.

Arthur P. Grollman, professor, Department of Pharmacology and Toxicology, Stony Brook University Medical School, Stony Brook, N.Y.; in-person interview May 5, 2012, and multiple e-mail exchanges.

Mark Schiffman, senior investigator, Division of Cancer Epidemiology and Genetics, National Cancer Institute, Bethesda, Md.; telephone interview, March 25, 2014.

Richard M. Sharpe, group leader, MRC Center for Reproductive Health, University of Edinburgh, Scotland; multiple e-mail exchanges, August 21, 25, and 30, 2014.

Robert E. Tarone, biostatistics director, International Epidemiology Institute, Rockville, Md.; in-person interview December, 2014, and multiple e-mail exchanges.

Allen Wilcox, principal investigator, Reproductive Epidemiology Group, National Institute of Environmental Health Sciences, Research Triangle Park, Durham, N.C.; October 20, 2014.

Mary S. Wolff, Professor, Departments of Preventive Medicine, Oncological Sciences, Mount Sinai Medical Center, New York, N.Y.; September 30, 2014.

# NOTES

## PREFACE

1. Bienkowsky B. BPA may prompt more fat deposition in the human body. *Scientific American* 2015 May 29. http://www.scientificamerican.com/article/bpa-may-prompt-more-fat-in-the-human-body/.

2. Stacy SL et al. Perinatal outcomes and unconventional natural gas operations in southwest Pennsylvania. *PLoS ONE* 2015 June 3. doi:10.1371/journal.pone.0126425, http://journals.plos.org/plosone/article?id=10.1371/journal.pone.0126425.

3. Goldberg P. Peers puzzled by Herberman's stance on cell phone while believers rally. *Cancer Letter* 2008;34, Aug. 1.

4. Taubes G. Diet advice that ignores hunger. *New York Times* 2015 Aug. 29.

5. Collins H. *Are We All Scientific Experts Now?* Malden, Mass.: Polity Press, 2014.

6. American Institute for Cancer Research. New survey: U.S. beliefs about cancer risk put fear before facts. 2015 Feb. 4. http://www.aicr.org/press/press-releases/2015/new-survey-us-beliefs-about-cancer-risk-put-fear-before-facts.html.

7. Taubes G. Epidemiology faces its limits. *Science* 1995;269:164–69.

8. Alberts B, Kirschner MW, Tilghman S, Varmus H. Rescuing biomedical research from its systematic flaws. *Proceedings of the National Academy of Sciences USA* 2014;111:5773–77; Landis SC et al. A call for transparent reporting to optimize the predictive value of preclinical research. *Nature* 2012;490:187–91.

9. Mooney C, Kirshenbaum G. *Unscientific America: How Scientific Illiteracy Threatens Our Future.* New York: Basic Books, 2009; Specter M. *Denialism: How Irrational*

*Thinking Hinders Scientific Progress, Harms the Planet, and Threatens Our Lives.* New York: Penguin, 2009; Shermer M. *The Believing Brain: From Ghosts and Gods to Politics and Conspiracies—How We Construct Beliefs and Reinforce Them as Truths.* New York: Times Books, 2011; Collins H. *Are We All Scientific Experts Now?* Malden, Mass.: Polity Press 2014; Offit P. *Autism's False Prophets: Bad Science, Risky Medicine, and the Search for a Cure.* New York: Columbia University Press, 2010; Mnookin S. *The Panic Virus: The True Story Behind the Vaccine-Autism Controversy.* New York: Simon and Schuster, 2012.

10. Morabia A. *Enigmas of Health and Disease: How Epidemiology Helps Unravel Scientific Mysteries.* New York: Columbia University Press, 2014; Bracken MB, *Risk, Chance, and Causation: Investigating the Origins and Treatment of Disease.* New Haven, Conn.: Yale University Press, 2013.

11. Kabat GC. *Hyping Health Risks: Environmental Hazards in Daily Life and the Science of Epidemiology.* New York: Columbia University Press, 2008.

## 1. THE ILLUSION OF VALIDITY AND
## THE POWER OF "NEGATIVE THINKING"

1. Dyson F. How to dispel your illusions, review of Daniel Kahneman, *Thinking, Fast and Slow. New York Review of Books* 2011 Dec. 22.

2. Mangel M, Samaniego F. Abraham Wald's work on aircraft survivability. *Journal of the American Statistical Association* 1984;79:259–67.

3. Ibid., 267.

4. Wald's insight is reminiscent of techniques that artists have long used to free themselves from the rote and therefore deadening habits that we all fall into. We are so used to the objects around us—the human figure, a chair—that it is difficult not to substitute our idea of the figure or chair for what is actually there. One trick artists use to circumvent these preconceptions is to draw what is *not* the figure or *not* the chair—what is referred to as the "negative space" surrounding the object.

When I told the story about Abraham Wald in a *Forbes* column (http://www.forbes.com/sites/geoffreykabat/2013/01/17/making-room-for-the-unseen-in-tackling-complex-problems/), an immunologist colleague, Lawrence Silbart of the University of Connecticut, wrote to me, "I had never heard about this before! This is of course how our immune repertoire is shaped. We subtract out self-reactive lymphocytes while they are immature and can't do any harm. Thus, only lymphocytes that react with other shapes (i.e., foreign intruders) are allowed to reach maturity. Presumably this system evolved since our immune systems can't anticipate what these new shapes are going to look like (since new pathogens emerge and old ones evolve) . . . so it's nature's Wald."

5. Kahneman D. *Thinking Fast and Slow.* New York: Farrar, Straus, and Giroux, 2011; Taleb NN. *Fooled by Randomness: The Hidden Role of Chance in Life and in the Markets.* New York: Random House, 2005; Tetlock P. *Expert Political Judgment: How Good Is It? How Can We Know?* Princeton, N.J.: Princeton University Press, 2006.

6. Goldacre B. *Bad Science*. London: Harper Perennial, 2008; Park R, *Voodoo Science: The Road from Foolishness to Fraud*. New York: Oxford University Press, 2000; Feynman R, Cargo cult science. http://en.wikipedia.org/wiki/Cargo_cult_science; Langmuir I. Pathological science. Transcribed and ed. RN Hall. *Physics Today* 1989 Oct.; Ames B, Gold LS. Paraselsus to parascience: the environment cancer distraction. *Mutation Research* 2000;447:3–13.

7. Watson JD. *The Double Helix*. New York: Signet Books, 1968; Darwin C. *The Origin of Species*. Middlesex, UK: Penguin Books, 1970; Thomas L. *Lives of a Cell: Notes of a Biology Watcher*. New York: Viking, 1974; Wilson EO. *Sociobiology*. Cambridge, Mass.: Belknap Press of Harvard University Press, 1975; Dawkins R. *The Selfish Gene*. Oxford: Oxford University Press, 1976; Rhodes R. *Deadly Feasts: Tracking the Secrets of a Terrifying New Plague*. New York: Simon and Schuster, 1997; Skloot R. *The Immortal Life of Henrietta Lacks*. New York: Broadway Books, 2010; Quammen D. *The Chimp and the River: How AIDS Emerged from an African Forest*. New York: Random House, 2015; Quammen D. *Spillover: Animal Infections and the Next Human Pandemic*. New York: Norton, 2012.

## 2. SPLENDORS AND MISERIES OF ASSOCIATIONS

1. Hormann AM et al. Holding thermal receipt paper and eating food afterward using hand sanitizer results in high serum bioactive and urine total levels of bisphenol A (BPA). *PLoS ONE* 2014 Oct. 22. doi:10.1371/journal.pone.0110509.

2. Associated Press. American Ebola doc: "I'm thrilled to be alive." *New York Times* 2014 Aug. 21.

3. I am referring to the paper by Andrew Wakefield published in the *Lancet* in 1998 claiming that there is a link between administration of the measles, mumps, and rubella vaccine and the appearance of autism and bowel disease in children. Twelve years later, owing to the efforts of a persistent investigative journalist, the work was shown to be fraudulent and the paper was retracted.

4. Centers for Disease Control and Prevention. U.S. Multi-state measles outbreak 2014–2015. http://www.cdc.gov/measles/multi-state-outbreak.html; Nagourney A, Goodnough A. Measles cases linked to Disneyland rise, and debate over vaccinations intensifies. *New York Times* 2014 Jan. 21; Xia R, Lin RG. Measles outbreak at 149 cases in eight states, Canada and Mexico. *Los Angeles Times* 2015 Feb. 20.

5. Satel SL. Will the F.D.A. kill off e-cigs (op-ed). *New York Times* 2015 Jan. 18; Fairchild AL, Bayer R. Smoke and fire over e-cigarettes. *Science* 2015;347:375–76.

6. Centers for Disease Control and Prevention. CDC estimates of foodborne illness in the United States 2014. http://www.cdc.gov/foodborneburden/.

7. Offit P. *Do You Believe in Magic? The Sense and Nonsense of Alternative Medicine*. New York: Harper, 2013; Navarro VJ et al. Liver injury from herbals and dietary supplements in the U.S.—drug-induced liver injury network. *Hepatology* 2014 60(4):1399–1408. doi:10.1002/hep.27317. Epub 2014 Aug. 25.

8. Geller AI et al. Emergency department visits for adverse events related to dietary supplements. *New England Journal of Medicine* 2015;15(373):1531–40. doi:10.1056/NEJMsa1504267.

9. Patel CJ, Cullen MR, Ioannidis JPA, Butte AJ. Systematic evaluation of environmental factors: persistent pollutants and nutrients correlated with serum lipids. *International Journal of Epidemiology* 2012;41:828–43.

10. Konkel L. Data Stretching back to 1959 may explain link between environment and breast cancer. *Scientific American* 2015 Apr. http://www.scientificamerican.com/article/data-stretching-back-to-1959-may-explain-link-between-environment-and-breast-cancer/; Cohn BA et al. DDT exposure in utero and breast cancer. *Journal of Endocrinology and Metabolism* 2015. doi:10.1210/jc.2015–1841.

11. Young SS, Karr A. Deming, data, and observational studies: a process out of control and needing fixing. *Significance* 2011;8:116–20. http://onlinelibrary.wiley.com/doi/10.1111/j.1740–9713.2011.00506.x/abstract.

12. World Cancer Research Fund/American Institute for Cancer Research. *Food, Nutrition, Physical Activity, and the Prevention of Cancer.* 2007.

13. Schoenfeld JD, Ioannidis JP. Is everything we eat associated with cancer? A systematic cookbook review. *American Journal of Clinical Nutrition* 2013;97:127–34. doi:10.3945/ajcn.112.047142. Epub 2012 Nov. 28.

14. Taubes G. Epidemiology faces its limits. *Science* 1995;269:164–69; Kabat GC. *Hyping Health Risks: Environmental Hazards in Everyday Life and the Science of Epidemiology.* New York: Columbia University Press, 2008; Boffetta P, McLaughlin JK, La Vecchia C, Tarone RE, Lipworth L, Blot WJ. False positive results in cancer epidemiology: a plea for epidemiologic modesty. *Journal of the National Cancer Institute* 2008;100:988–95; Young, Karr. Deming, data and observational studies; Bhopal R. Seven mistakes and potential solutions in epidemiology, including a call for a World Council of Epidemiology and Causality. *Emerging Themes in Epidemiology* 2009;6:6. doi:10.1186/1742–7622–6-6; Rothman KJ. Six persistent research misconceptions. *Journal of General Internal Medicine* 2014;29:1060–64. doi:10.1007/s11606–013–2755-z.

15. Ioannidis JPA. Why most research findings are false. *PLoS Medicine* 2005;2:e124. doi:10.1371/journal.pmed.0020124.

16. Freedman DH. Lies, damned lies, and medical science. *Atlantic* 2010 Nov. 20.

17. Ioannidis JPA. Contradicted and initially stronger effects in highly cited clinical research. *JAMA* 2005;294:218–28.

18. Tsilidis KT, Papatheordorou SI, Evangelou E, Ioannidis JPA. Evaluation of excess statistical significance in meta-analyses of 98 biomarker associations with cancer risk. *Journal of the National Cancer Institute* 2012;104:1867–75.

19. Ioannidis JP. How to make more published research true. *PLoS Medicine* 2014;11(10):e1001747. doi:10.1371/journal.pmed.1001747. eCollection 2014.

20. Hill AB. The environment and disease: association or causation? *Proceedings of the Royal Society of Medicine* 1965;58:295–300.

21. Rothman KJ, Greenland S. Causation and causal inference in epidemiology. *American Journal Public Health* 2005;95:S144–S150. doi:10.2105/AJPH.2004.059204; Gee

D. Late lessons from early warnings: toward realism and precaution with endocrine-disrupting substances. *Environmental Health Perspectives* 2006;114 Suppl.:152–60.

22. Phillips CV, Goodman KJ. The missed lessons of Sir Austin Bradford Hill. *Epidemiologic Perspectives and Innovations.* 2004;1:3. http://www.ncbi.nlm.nih.gov /pubmed/15507128.

23. Rothman, Greenland. Causation and causal inference in epidemiology.

24. Ibid.

25. Ibid.

26. Ibid.

27. Kabat G. After 40 years of research, what do we know about preventing breast cancer? *Forbes* 2013 Feb. 24.

28. "Circular epidemiology can be defined as the continuation of specific types of epidemiologic studies beyond the point of reasonable doubt of the true existence of an important association or the absence of such an association." Kuller L. Circular epidemiology. *American Journal of Epidemiology* 1999;150:897–903.

29. Savitz D. The etiology of epidemiologic perseveration: when enough is enough. *Epidemiology* 2010;21:281–83. doi:10.1097/EDE.0b013e3181d77b5f.

30. Platt JR. Strong inference. *Science* 1964;146:347–53.

31. Chamberlin TC. The method of multiple working hypotheses. *Science* 1890;15:92–96.

32. "When multiple hypotheses become coupled to strong inference, the scientific search becomes an emotional powerhouse as well as an intellectual one." Platt. Strong inference.

33. Ibid.

## 3. WHEN RISK GOES VIRAL: BIASES AND BANDWAGONS

1. Latour B. *We Never Have Been Modern*, trans. Catherine Porter. Cambridge, Mass.: Harvard University Press, 1993.

2. Kabat GC. *Hyping Health Risks: Environmental Hazards in Daily Life and the Science of Epidemiology*. New York: Columbia University Press, 2008.

3. Chang K. Debate continues on hazards of electromagnetic waves. *New York Times* 2014 July 7.

4. "Even today, though the caveat that the occurrence of two events (association) does not indicate causality is widely recognized, Hume's identification of this limitation in the search for causal relationships is often ignored. The seduction of inductive reasoning is a trap that easily catches the unwary." Rabins PV. *The Why of Things: Causality in Science, Medicine, and Life*. New York: Columbia University Press, 2013, 14.

5. Jordan VC. Avoiding the bad and enhancing the good of soy supplements in breast cancer (editorial). *Journal of the National Cancer Institute* 2014;106:dju233. doi:10.1093/jnci/dju233.

6. Quoted in Taubes G. Epidemiology faces its limits. *Science* 1995;269:164–69.

7. Boffetta P, McLaughlin JK, La Vecchia C, Tarone RE, Lipworth L, Blot WJ. False-positive results in cancer epidemiology: a plea for epidemiologic modesty. *Journal of the National Cancer Institute* 2008;100:988–95; McLaughlin JK, Tarone RE. False positives in cancer epidemiology. *Cancer Epidemiology Biomarkers and Prevention* 2013;22:11–15. doi:10.1158/1055-9965.EPI-12-0995; Ioannidis JPA. Why most published research findings are false. *PLoS Medicine* 2005. doi:10.1371/journal.pmed.0020124; Kabat. *Hyping Health Risks*; Collins FS, Tabak LA. NIH plans to enhance reproducibility. *Nature* 2014;505:612–13; Dawn K et al. Systematic review of the empirical evidence of study publication bias and outcome reporting bias. *PLoS ONE* 2008;3:e3081.

8. Kabat. *Hyping Health Risks*.

9. Kabat G. Having it both ways on what causes cancer: IARC's flawed paradigm. *Forbes* 2015 Nov. 19. http://www.forbes.com/sites/geoffreykabat/2015/11/19/having-it-both-ways-on-what-causes-cancer/.

10. According to IARC's own "Preamble" to the monographs series setting out its mission, "A cancer 'hazard' is an agent that is capable of causing cancer *under some circumstances*, while a cancer 'risk' is an estimate of the carcinogenic effects expected from exposure to a cancer hazard" (emphasis added). The preamble goes on to state, "The Monographs are an exercise in evaluating cancer hazards, despite the historical presence of the word 'risks' in the title. The distinction between hazard and risk is important, and the Monographs identify cancer hazards *even when risks are very low at current exposure levels*, because new uses or unforeseen exposures could engender risks that are significantly higher" (emphasis added). http://monographs.iarc.fr/ENG/Preamble/CurrentPreamble.pdf.

11. Plummer B. The bacon freak-out: why the WHO's cancer warnings cause so much confusion. *Vox* 2015 Oct. 26. http://www.vox.com/2015/10/26/9617928/iarc-cancer-risk-carcinogenic.

12. Gupta N, Stopfer M. Negative results need airing too. *Nature* 2011;470. doi:10.1038/470039a; Yong E. Replication studies: bad copy. *Nature* 2012 485:298–300. doi:10.1038/485298a; Nyhan B. To get more out of science, show the rejected research. *New York Times* 2014 Sept. 18.

13. The magnifying glass effect is very much in line with the kinds of biases described by Kahneman and Tversky, especially the availability heuristic.

14. Slovic P, ed. *The Perception of Risk*. London: Earthscan, 2000.

15. Phalen R. California Air Resources Board PM 2.5 Mortality Symposium, Sacramento Calif., Feb. 26, 2010. https://www.youtube.com/watch?v=CIGFgyhaw20.

16. Cope MB, Allison DB. White hat bias: examples of its presence in obesity research and a call for renewed commitment to faithfulness in research reporting. *International Journal of Obesity* 2010;34:84–88; Atkinson RL, Macdonald I. White hat bias: the need for authors to have the spin stop with them (editorial). *International Journal of Obesity* 2010;34:83.

17. Kabat G. The crisis of peer review. *Forbes* 2015 Nov. 23. http://www.forbes.com/sites/geoffreykabat/2015/11/23/the-crisis-of-peer-review/.

18. Wakefield AJ et al. Ileal-lymphoid-nodular hyperplasia, non-specific colitis, and pervasive developmental disorder in children. *Lancet* 1998 Feb 28;351(9103):637–41;

retraction in *Lancet* 2010 Feb 6;375(9713):445; partial retraction in Murch SH et al. *Lancet* 2004 Mar 6;363(9411):750; Deer B. How the case against MMR was fixed. *BMJ* 2011;342. doi:http://dx.doi.org/10.1136/bmj.c5347.

19. Rothman KJ. Conflict of interest: the new McCarthyism in science. *Journal of the American Medical Association* 1993;269:2782–84; Conflict of interest policies: protecting readers or censoring authors? In reply. *Journal of the American Medical Association* 1993;270:2684.

20. Trinquart L, Johns DM, Galea S. Why do we think we know what we know? A metaknowledge analysis of the salt controversy. *International Journal of Epidemiology* 2016;45:251–60.

21. Feynman R. Cargo cult science: some remarks on science, pseudoscience, and learning how to not fool yourself. Commencement address, California Institute of Technology, 1974. http://calteches.library.caltech.edu/51/2/CargoCult.htm.

22. Quoted in Taubes. Epidemiology faces its limits.

23. The precautionary principle. https://commons.wikimedia.org.

24. Sunstein CR. Beyond the precautionary principle. *John M. Olin Law & Economics Working Paper* no. 149 (2nd series), *Public Law and Legal Theory Working Paper* no. 38 (January 2003): 8. http://ssrn.com/abstract_id=307098 p. 8.

25. Ibid., 2. Sunstein goes so far as to argue that the precautionary principle is useless because "it leads in no direction at all. The reason is that risks of one kind or another are on all sides of regulatory choices and it is therefore impossible, in most real-world cases, to avoid running afoul of the principle" (42). He explains the enormous appeal of the principle and its incorporation into legal and political discourse by its conformity with cognitive biases, such as loss aversion and the availability heuristic (5–7).

26. To name just a few instances: IARC's questionable assessments of cells phones, coffee, formaldehyde, and glyphosate; NIEHS's program supporting research on BPA; and DOE's and NIEHS's earlier program on EMFs.

27. Trinquart, Johns, Galea. Why do we think we know what we know?

28. Kahneman D, Tversky A. Judgment under uncertainty: heuristics and biases. *Science* 1974;185:1124–31; Kahneman D. *Thinking Fast and Slow*. New York: Farrar, Straus, and Giroux, 2011.

29. Kuran T, Sunstein CR. Availability cascades and risk regulation. *Working Paper Series*, 685. http://www.law.uchicago.edu/Lawecon/index.html, and at *Public Law and Legal Theory Working Paper Series*. http://www.law.uchicago.edu/academics/publiclaw/index.html, and Social Science Research Network Electronic Paper Collection. http://ssrn.com/abstract_id=1019644.

30. Ibid.

31. Ibid., 691–97. George Johnson situates the Love Canal incident in the context of ideas about cancer and the environment that were prevalent in the 1970s, in *The Cancer Chronicles: Unlocking Medicine's Deepest Mystery*. New York: Knopf, 2013.

32. Kuran, Sunstein. Availability cascades and risk regulation, 713.

33. Ibid., 716–17, 726.

## 4. DO CELL PHONES CAUSE BRAIN CANCER? A TALE OF TWO SCIENCES

1. Park RL. Cellular telephones and cancer: how should science respond? *Journal of the National Cancer Institute* 2001;93:166–67. Resorting to a form of magical thinking, Reynard went on to say, "The tumor was exactly in the pattern of the antenna." Mukherjee S, Do cellphones cause brain cancer? *New York Times* magazine 2011 April 13.

2. Linet MS, Inskip PD. Cellular (mobile) telephone use and cancer risk. *Reviews on Environmental Health* 2010;25:51–55.

3. Park. Cellular telephones and cancer.

4. For an account of the rise and fall of the controversy surrounding the health effects of exposure to EMFs, see Kabat GC. *Hyping Health Risks: Environmental Hazards in Daily Life and the Science of Epidemiology*. New York: Columbia University Press, 2008, chap. 4.

5. Rothman KJ. Health effects of mobile telephones (editorial). *Epidemiology* 2009;20(5):653–55.

6. American Cancer Society. *Cancer Facts and Figures 2014*. http://www.cancer.org /research/cancerfactsstatistics/cancerfactsfigures2014/.

7. Ahlbom A, Green A, Kheifets L, Savitz D, Swerdlow A. Epidemiology of health effects of radiofrequency exposure. *Environmental Health Perspectives* 2004;112:1741–54; Linet, Inskip. Cellular (mobile) telephone use.

8. Ahlbom et al. Epidemiology of health effects.

9. Ibid.

10. Kabat. *Hyping Health Risks*, chap. 4.

11. INTERPHONE Study Group. Brain tumours risk in relation to mobile telephone use: results of the INTERPHONE international case-control study. *International Journal of Epidemiology* 2010;39:675–94.

12. Ahlbom A, Feychting M, Green A, Kheifets L, Savitz DA, Swerdlow AJ, International Commission for Non-Ionizing Radiation Protection (ICNIRP) Standing Committee on Epidemiology. Epidemiologic evidence on mobile phones and tumor risk: a review. *Epidemiology* 2009;20:639–52.

13. Repacholi MH et al. Systematic review of wireless phone use and brain cancer and other head tumors (review). *Bioelectromagnetics* 2012;33:187–206; Lagorio S, Röösli M. Mobile phone use and risk of intracranial tumors: a consistency analysis. *Bioelectromagnetics* 2014;35:79–90; Scientific Committee on Emerging and Newly Identified Health Risks (SCENIHR). *Potential Health Effects of Exposure to Electromagnetic Fields (EMF)*. 2015, 72–84.

14. Hardell L, Carlberg M. Mobile phones, cordless phones and the risk for brain tumours. *International Journal of Oncology* 2009;35:5–17; Hardell L, Carlberg M, Hansson MK. Pooled analysis of case-control studies on malignant brain tumours and use of mobile and cordless phones including living and deceased subjects. *International Journal of Oncology* 2011;38:1465–74.

15. Ahlbom A, Feychting M. Mobile telephones and brain tumors (editorial). *BMJ* 2011;343.d6605. doi:10.1136/bmj.d6605.

16. Deltour I, Johansen C, Auvinen A, Feychting M, Klaeboe L, Schüz J. Time trends in brain tumor incidence rates in Denmark, Finland, Norway, and Sweden, 1974–2003. *Journal of the National Cancer Institute* 2009;101:1721–24; Deltour IU et al. Mobile phone use and incidence of glioma in the Nordic countries 1979–2008: consistency check. *Epidemiology* 2012;23:301–307; De Vocht F, Burstyn I, Cherrie JW. Time trends (1998–2007) in brain cancer incidence rates in relation to mobile phone use in England. *Bioelectromagnetics* 2011;32:334–39; Little MP et al. Mobile phone use and glioma risk: comparison of epidemiological study results with incidence trends in the United States. *BMJ* 2012;344:e114. doi:10.1136/bmj.e1147.

17. Repacholi et al. Systematic review of wireless phone use; Lagorio, Röösli. Mobile phone use.

18. http://www.bioinitiative.org.

19. Goldberg P. Peers puzzled by Herberman's stance on cell phone while believers rally. *Cancer Letter* 2008;34, Aug. 1.

20. *Cell Phones and Brain Tumors: 15 Reasons for Concern.* http://www.radiation research.org/pdfs/reasons_us.pdf; Environmental Working Group. *Cell Phone Radiation: Science Review on Cancer Risks and Children's Health.* http://static.ewg.org/reports/2012 /cellphones/2009-cellphoneradiation-fullreport.pdf?_ga=1.222126232.1202499323 .1425218899.

21. *Cell Phones and Brain Tumors.*

22. Ibid.; Environmental Working Group. *Cell Phone Radiation.*

23. Khurana VG, Teo C, Kundi M, Hardell L, Carlberg M. Cell phones and brain tumors: a review including the long-term epidemiologic data. *Surgical Neurology* 2009;72:205–14; discussion 214–15. Epub 2009 Mar. 27.

24. Myung SK et al. Mobile phone use and risk of tumors: a meta-analysis. *Journal of Clinical Oncology* 2009;27:5565–72. Epub 2009 Oct. 13.

25. Davis D. Brain cancer and cell phones: the jury is still out. *Huffington Post* 2009 Dec. 7. http://www.huffingtonpost.com/devra-davis-phd/brain-cancer-and-cell -pho_b_379601.html.

26. Kabat. *Hyping Health Risks*, chap. 3.

27. Davis DL, Bradlow HL, Wolff M, Woodruff T, Hoel DG, Anton-Culver H. Medical hypothesis: xenoestrogens as preventable causes of breast cancer. *Environmental Health Perspectives* 1993;101:372–77.

28. Davis. Brain cancer and cell phones; Davis D. *Disconnect: The Truth About Cell Phone Radiation, What the Industry Has Done to Hide It, and How to Protect Your Family.* New York: Dutton, 2010.

29. Davis D. Cell phones and brain cancer: the real story. *Huffington Post* 2010 May 22. http://www.huffingtonpost.com/devra-davis-phd/cell-phones-and-brain -can_b_585992.html.

30. Sunstein CR. *Laws of Fear.* Cambridge: Cambridge University Press, 2005; Cross FR. Paradoxical perils of the precautionary principle. *Washington and Lee Law Review* 1996;53:851–925.

31. Sunstein. *Laws of Fear*; Cross. Paradoxical perils.

32. *Bioinitiative 2012*, Summary for the Public (2014 Supplement). http://www
.bioinitiative.org/report/wp-content/uploads/pdfs/sec01_2012_summary_for_public.pdf.

33. Davis. Cell phones and brain cancer; Davis. *Disconnect.*

34. The INTERPHONE Study Group. Brain tumours risk.

35. Not surprisingly, print and web news stories—I counted ninety hits from my
"Google alert" for "INTERPHONE study" between May 15 and August 14, 2010—reported
these ambiguous findings in a variety of ways. To some, this largest of studies found no
evidence of a hazard, while to others the study provided evidence of a "cancer link." It
is noteworthy, however, that a large proportion of news stories correctly highlighted the
lack of any clear-cut evidence of an effect.

36. Saracci R, Samet J. Commentary: call me on my mobile phone . . . or better not?—a look at the Interphone study results. *International Journal of Epidemiology*
2010;39:695–698.

37. Frei P, Poulsen AH, Johansen C, Olsen JH, Steding-Jessen M, Schüz J. Use of
mobile phones and brain tumors: update of Danish cohort study. *BMJ* 2011;343:d6387.

38. Inskip PD, Hoover RN, Devesa SS. Brain cancer incidence trends in relation to
cellular telephone use in the United States. *Neuro-Oncology* 2010;12:1147–51.

39. Deltour et al. Time trends in brain tumor incidence rates; Deltour et al. Mobile
phone use and incidence of glioma.

40. De Vocht F, Burstyn I, Cherrie JW. Time trends (1998–2007).

41. Little et al. Mobile phone use and glioma risk.

42. SCENIHR. Potential health effects of exposure, 86.

43. Ibid., 101.

44. Moulder JE, Foster KR, Erdreich LS, McNamee JP. Mobile phones, mobile
phone base stations and cancer: a review. *International Journal of Radiation Biology*
2005;81:189–203.

45. Adair RK. Biophysical limits on athermal effects of RF and microwave radiation. *Bioelectromagnetics*. 2003;24:39–48.

46. Volkow ND et al. Effects of cell phone radiofrequency signal exposure on brain
glucose metabolism. *JAMA* 2011;305:808–13. doi:10.1001/jama.2011.186.

47. Letters in response to Volkow et al.: Kosowsky A, Swanson E , Gerjuoy E. Cell
phone activation and brain glucose metabolism; Davis CC; Nordström C-H; Volkow
ND, Tomasi D, Vaska P. *JAMA* 2011;305:2066–68.

48. Kwon MS et al. GSM mobile phone radiation suppresses brain glucose metabolism. *Journal of Cerebral Blood Flow & Metabolism* 2011;31:2293–2301.

49. Baan R et al. Carcinogenicity of radiofrequency magnetic fields. *Lancet Oncology* 2011;12:624–26.

50. Boffetta P, McLaughlin JK, La Vecchia C, Tarone RE, Lipworth L, Blot WJ.
False-positive results in cancer epidemiology: a plea for epistemological modesty. *Jour-
nal of the National Cancer Institute* 2008 July 16;100(14):988–95. doi:10.1093/jnci/djn191.
Epub 2008 Jul 8; Boffetta P, McLaughlin JK, La Vecchia C, Tarone RE, Lipworth L,
Blot WJ. A further plea for adherence to the principles underlying science in general
and the epidemiologic enterprise in particular. *International Journal of Epidemiology*

2009 38(3):678–79. doi:10.1093/ije/dyn362; McLaughlin JK, Tarone RE. False positives in cancer epidemiology. *Cancer Epidemiology Biomarkers and Prevention* 2012;22:11–15; Kabat G. How activism distorts the assessment of health risks. *Forbes* 2012 Nov. 20; Kabat G. Behind the World Health Organization's "cancerous" pronouncement on cell phones. *Forbes* 2011 Aug. 23. http://www.forbes.com/sites/realspin/2011/08/23/world -health-organization-cancerous-cell-phones/.

51. World Health Organization. International Agency for Research on Cancer. IARC Monographs on the Evaluation of Carcinogenic Risks to Humans: Preamble, Lyon, France, 2006. http://monographs.iarc.fr/ENG/Preamble/CurrentPreamble.pdf.

52. Wiedemann PM, Boerner FU, Repacholi MH. Do people understand IARC's 2B categorization of RF fields from cell phones? *Bioelectromagnetics* 2014;35:373–78.

53. According to Dr. Vijayalaxmi, who was a member of the IARC Working Group on cell phones, in issuing its report IARC wanted to send a message that we still have limited information about the possible effects of prolonged and heavy use of cell phones, especially among users who start as children and adolescents. She is comfortable with the classification and thinks that it will be an "eye-opener for people who abuse the technology, which is meant for benefit, not for overuse and abuse." Quoted in Kabat. Behind the World Health Organization's "cancerous" pronouncement."

54. Associated Press. Cellphones a "possible" carcinogen—like coffee. *Seattle Times* 2011 June 1. http://www.columbiatribune.com/news/who-panel-lists-cellphones-as-possible-carcinogen-like-coffee/article_75f0a55f-4457-5b8c-8fb7-287010d42027.html.

55. The Cohort Study of Mobile Phone Use and Health (COSMOS) is a cohort study of mobile phone use and health that is in the process of recruiting approximately 250,000 men and women in Denmark, Finland, Sweden, Netherlands, and Great Britain. Participants will be followed for at least twenty-five years, and exposure information will be collected via both questionnaires and objective data from telecommunications providers, which represents an improvement over previous studies. Outcomes will be determined by linkage to disease registries. However, there is a serious problem confronting studies undertaken at this point in time—that is, that exposure to RF from cell phones and other wireless appliances is nearly ubiquitous, and this reduces the ability to detect an effect of exposure.

## 5. HORMONAL CONFUSION: THE CONTESTED SCIENCE OF ENDOCRINE DISRUPTION

1. Carlsen E, Giwercman A, Keiding N, Skakkebaek NE. Evidence for decreasing quality of semen during past 50 years. *BMJ* 1992;305:609–13.

2. Colborn T, Dumanski D, Myers JP. *Our Stolen Future*. New York: Plume Books, 1997; Krimsky S, *Hormonal Chaos: The Scientific and Social Origins of the Environmental Endocrine Hypothesis*. Baltimore: Johns Hopkins University Press, 2000.

3. Krimsky. *Hormonal Chaos*, 48–51.

4. Herbst AL, Ulfelder H, Poskanzer DC. Adenocarcinoma of the vagina. Association of maternal stilbestrol therapy with tumor appearance in young women. *New England Journal of Medicine* 1971 Apr. 15;284(15):878–81.

5. The central importance of the DES experience as a model for those studying the effects of chemicals in the environment is conveyed by John McLachlan, a scientist who has spent his career studying the biological mechanisms by which early exposure to chemicals, including DES, might set the stage for future disease. In 2001 he wrote, "The universe of chemicals 'endowed with estrogenic properties' has grown enormously in the last 30 years. Environmental compounds have also been discovered that are anti-estrogens and anti-androgens. Species as diverse as snails and humans are thought to be affected by endocrine disruption. It is all the more remarkable that the principles used to establish this growing list of hormonally active chemicals were, and continue to be, based on the potent synthetic estrogen DES and the clinical experience first reported 30 years ago." McLachlan JA, Newbold RR, Burow ME, Li SF. From malformations to molecular mechanisms in the male: three decades of research on endocrine disrupters. *APMIS* 2001;109:263–72.

6. Environmental History Timeline. http://www.environmentalhistory.org/.

7. Higginson J. Cancer and the environment: Higginson speaks out. *Science* 1979;205:1363–64.

8. Colborn, Dumanski, Myers. *Our Stolen Future*, 259–68; Krimsky. *Hormonal Chaos*, 24–29. For good early discussions of the endocrine disruption hypothesis, see Hollander D. Environmental effects on reproductive health: the endocrine disruption hypothesis. *Family Planning Perspectives* 1997;29:82–89; Baker VA, Endocrine disrupter—testing strategies to assess human hazard. *Toxicology in Vitro* 2001;15:413–19.

9. Sharpe RM, Skakkebaek NE. Are oestrogens involved in falling sperm counts and disorders of the male reproductive tract? *Lancet* 1993;341:1392–95. Commenting on this hypothesis paper in 2014, Sharpe had the following to say: "It has become a citation classic (hint: to get high citations, never include data!). Yet time and further research has proved that the hypothesis is fundamentally flawed, because human foetal Leydig cells do not express full-length oestrogen receptor alpha (ESR1) as do rodent foetal Lyedig cells, and it is ESR1 that mediates the adverse effects of estrogens on the foetal testis." Sharpe RM. Lessons learned from andrology. *Andrology* 2014;2:652–55.

10. Boisen KA, Main KM, Rajpert-de-Meyts E, Skakkebaek NE. Are male reproductive disorders a common entity? *Annals of the New York Academy of Sciences* 2001;948:90–99.

11. PubMed citations "environmental endocrine disruptors." http://www.ncbi.nlm.nih.gov/pubmed/?term=environmental+endocrine+disruptors.

12. Krimsky. *Hormonal Chaos*, 105.

13. Ibid., 2, 3. It's worth noting that the two successful hypotheses cited by Krimsky were highly focused and specific and led to the identification of a specific mechanism that added clear-cut and important new knowledge. In contrast, the endocrine disruption hypothesis was all-encompassing, incorporating countless distinct phenomena and exposures, and innumerable potential mechanisms. Rather than a specific hypothesis, it was really a vast program of research.

14. Safe HS. Environmental and dietary estrogens and human health: is there a problem? *Environmental Health Perspectives* 1995;103:346–51; Safe HS. Is there an association between exposure to environmental estrogens and breast cancer? *Environmental Health Perspectives* 1997;105:675–78; Safe HS. Endocrine disruptors and human health—is there a problem? An update. *Environmental Health Perspectives* 2000;108:487–493; Joffe M. Are problems with male reproductive health caused by endocrine disruption? *Occupational and Environmental Medicine* 2001;58:281–87; Hollander. Environmental effects on reproductive health.

15. Particularly Richard Sharpe has embodied this.

16. Two such figures are Richard Sharpe and Stephen Safe.

17. Hollander. Environmental effects on reproductive health.

18. Ibid.

19. Ioannidis JAP. Contradicted and initially stronger effects in highly cited clinical research. *JAMA* 2005;294:218–28; Boffetta P, McLaughlin JK, La Vecchia C, Tarone RE, Lipworth L, Blot WJ. False positives in cancer epidemiology: a plea for epidemiologic modesty. *Journal of the National Cancer Institute* 2008;100:988–95; Kabat. *Hyping Health Risks.*

20. Safe. Environmental and dietary estrogens; Safe. Is there an association?; Safe. Endocrine disruptors and human health.

21. Hollander. Environmental effects on reproductive health.

22. Longnecker MP et al. An approach to assessment of endocrine disruption in the National Children's Study. *Environmental Health Perspectives* 2003;111:1691–97.

23. Colborn, Dumanski, Myers. *Our Stolen Future,* 67–69; Longnecker MP, Rogan WJ, Lucier G. The human health effects of DDT (dichlorodiphenyltrichloroethane) and PCBs (polychlorinated biphenyls) and an overview of organochlorines in public health. *Annual Review of Public Health* 1997;18:211–44.

24. Obaid Faroon, *Toxicological Profile on DDT.* Darby, Penn.: Diane Publishing, 2010. https://books.google.com/books/about/Toxicological_Profile_for_DDT_DDD_DDE _Up.html?id=qWs2ofoSm_4C&hl=en.

25. Wolff MS, Toniolo PG, Lee EW, Rivera M, Dubin N. Blood levels of organochlorine residues and risk of breast cancer. *Journal of the National Cancer Institute* 1993;85(8):648–52.

26. Hunter DJ, Kelsey KT. Pesticide residues and breast cancer: the harvest of a silent spring? *Journal of the National Cancer Institute* 1993;85:598–99.

27. MacMahon B. Pesticide residues and breast cancer? *Journal of the National Cancer Institute* 1994;86:572–73.

28. Lopez-Cervantes M et al. Dichlorodiphenyldichloroethane burden and breast cancer risk: a meta-analysis of the epidemiologic evidence. *Environmental Health Perspectives* 2004;112:207–14.

29. A more recent meta-analysis, which included forty-six studies, obtained a similar result. Ingber SZ, Buser MC, Pohl HR, Abadin HG, Murray HE, Scinicariello F. DDT/DDE and breast cancer: a meta-analysis. *Regulatory Toxicology and Pharmacology* 2013;67:421–33. doi:10.1016/j.yrtph.2013.08.021. Epub 2013 Sept. 8.

30. Institute of Medicine. *Breast Cancer and the Environment: A Life Course Approach*. Washington, D.C.: National Academies Press, 2012.

31. http://www.niehs.nih.gov/research/supported/dert/programs/breast-cancer /, accessed Dec. 1, 2014.

32. Joffe M. What has happened to human fertility? *Human Reproduction* 2010;25:295–307.

33. Ibid.

34. Kolata G. Sperm counts: some experts see a fall, others poor data. *New York Times* 1996 Mar. 19.

35. Ibid.

36. Ibid.

37. Joffe went on to comment that "an odd feature of this literature is the way it has been framed: the hypothesis has been of a global decline in sperm concentration, with an assumption that the level at any given time is the same in all parts of the world. . . . If this were true it would be unusual, possibly unique, in all epidemiology. This way of posing it means that any item of evidence tends to be regarded either as confirming or refuting a global decline, rather than providing information on the population from which the data were drawn." Joffe. What has happened to human fertility?, 296.

38. Fisch H. Declining worldwide sperm counts: disproving a myth. *Urologic Clinics of North America* 2008;35:137–46.

39. Ibid., 137.

40. Ibid.; Joffe. What has happened to human fertility?

41. Joffe M, Holmes J, Jensen TK, Keiding N, Best N. Time trends in biological fertility in Western Europe. *American Journal of Epidemiology* 2013;178:722–30.

42. Joffe, What has happened to human fertility?; Safe S. Clinical correlates of environmental endocrine disruptors. *Trends in Endocrinology and Metabolism* 2005;16:139–44.

43. Paulozzi LJ. International trends in rates of hypospadias and cryptorchidism. *Environmental Health Perspectives* 1999;107:297–302.

44. Fisch H, Hyun G, Hensle TW. Rising hypospadias rates: disproving a myth. *Journal of Pediatric Urology* 2010;6:37–39; Safe. Clinical correlates.

45. Joffe. What has happened to human fertility?, 302.

46. Dodds EC, Lawson W. Synthetic oestrogenic agents without a phenanthrene nucleus. *Nature* 1936;137:996–97.

47. The journalist Trevor Butterworth has chronicled the BPA saga since it became a high-profile story, explaining the scientific issues, pointing out the weaknesses of many published studies that received media attention, interviewing key researchers, and holding media coverage to account for its lax standards. *Forbes.com*. http://www.forbes .com/sites/trevorbutterworth/.

48. Nagel SC, vom Saal FS, Thayer KA, Dhar MG, Boechler M, Welshons WV. Relative binding affinity-serum modified access (RBA-SMA) assay predicts the relative in vivo bioactivity of the xenoestrogens bisphenol A and octylphenol. *Environmental Health Perspectives* 1997;105:70–76.

49. Goodman JE et al. Weight-of-evidence evaluation of reproductive and developmental effects of low doses of bisphenol A. *Critical Reviews in Toxicology* 2009;39(1): 1–75. doi:10.3109/10408440903279946.

50. Ibid.; Kamrin MA. The "low dose" hypothesis: validity and implications for human risk. *International Journal of Toxicology* 2007;26:13–23.

51. Rhomberg LR, Goodman JE. Low-dose and nonmonotonic dose-responses of endocrine disrupting chemicals: has the case been made? *Regulatory Toxicology and Pharmacology* 2012;64:130–33. Kamrin. The "low-dose" hypothesis.

52. vom Saal FS, Nagel SC, Timms BG, Welshons WV. Implications for human health of the extensive bisphenol A literature showing adverse effects at low doses: a response to attempts to mislead the public. *Toxicology* 2005;212:244–52. Tyl RW. Basic exploratory research versus guideline-compliant studies used for hazard evaluation and risk assessment: bisphenol A as a case study. *Environmental Health Perspectives* 2009;117:1644–51. doi:10.1289/chp.0900893.

53. Elswick BA, Welsh F, Janszen DB. Effect of different sampling designs on outcome of endocrine disruptor studies. *Reproductive Toxicology* 2000;14:359–67.

54. Ibid.; Kamrin. The "low dose" hypothesis; Owens JW, Chaney JG. Weighing the results of differing "low dose" studies of the mouse prostate by Nagel, Cagen, and Ashby: quantification of experimental power and statistical results. *Regulatory Toxicology and Pharmacology* 2005;43:194–202; Tyl. Basic exploratory research.

55. Teeguarden JG et al. Twenty-four hour human urine and serum profile of bisphenol A during high dietary exposure. *Toxicological Science* 2011;123:48–57.

56. Doerge DR, Twaddle NC, Woodling KA, Fisher JW. Pharmacokinetics of bisphenol A in neonatal and adult rhesus monkeys. *Toxicology and Applied Pharmacology* 2010 Oct 1;248(1):1–11. doi:10.1016/j.taap.2010.07.009. Epub 2010 Jul 23; Fisher JW, Twaddle NC, Vanlandingham M, Doerge DR. Pharmacokinetic modeling: prediction and evaluation of route dependent dosimetry of bisphenol A in monkeys with extrapolation to humans. *Toxicology and Applied Pharmacology* 2011 Nov. 15;257(1):122–36. doi:10.1016/j.taap.2011.08.026. Epub 2011 Sept. 2.

57. Teeguarden et al. Twenty-four hour human urine.

58. Teeguarden J, Hanson-Drury, Fisher JW, Doerge DR. Are typical serum BPA concentrations measurable and sufficient to be estrogenic in the general population? *Food and Chemical Toxicology* 2013;62:949–63.

59. Ibid.

60. Vandenberg LN et al. Regulatory decisions on endocrine disrupting chemicals should be based on the principles of endocrinology. *Reproductive Toxicology* 2013;38:1–15. doi:10.1016/j.reprotox.2013.02.002; Vom Saal FS, Welshons WV. Evidence that bisphenol A (BPA) can be accurately measured without contamination in human serum and urine and that BPA causes numerous hazards from multiple routes of exposure. *Molecular and Cellular Endocrinology* 2014;398:101–13. http://dx.doi.org/10.1016/j.mce.2014.09.028.

61. Bergman A, Heindel JJ, Jobling S, Kidd KA, Zoeller RT, eds. *Endocrine Disrupting Chemicals 2012: The State of the Science*. Geneva: World Health Organization

and United Nations Environment Programme, 2013. http://www.who.int/ceh/publications/endocrine/en/. Written by a group containing a number of endocrine disruption advocates, this three-hundred-page document presented an enormous amount of information, accompanied by graphs, charts, and maps, to dramatize the potential impact on wildlife and human health from exposure to endocrine disrupting chemicals worldwide. However, the document confused two issues: one that is not controversial and for which there is abundant, strong evidence—that is, effects of pollution on the environment in the broadest sense (ocean acidification, pollution of waterways with runoff, destruction of habitat, extinction of species, etc.); and one for which there is no clear or consistent evidence—namely, the effects of exposure to trace amounts of these chemicals on human health and development. This obliges the authors to imply that endocrine disruption *might* be playing a role in a wide range of health outcomes: cancers of the breast, prostate, testicles, and endometrium; birth defects; sperm count; fertility; and obesity. But they use selective citation to make their case and ignore evidence that does not support their thesis. The report trades on this basic confusion in its appeal to politicians and a concerned public. For systematic critiques of the *State of the Science* report, see Lamb JC IV et al. Critical comments on the WHO-UNEP State of the Science of Endocrine Disrupting Chemicals—2012. *Regulatory Toxicology and Pharmacology* 2014;69:22–40; Testai E, Galli CL, Dekant W, Marinovich M, Piersma AH, Sharpe RM. A plea for risk assessment of endocrine disrupting chemicals. *Toxicology* 2013;314:d51–59.

62. Dietrich D et al. Open letter to the European Commission: scientifically unfounded precaution drives European Commission's recommendation on EDC reduction, while defying common sense, well-established science, and risk assessment principles. *Food Chemistry and Toxicology* 2015;62:A1–A4.

63. Bergman A, et al. Science and policy on endocrine disrupters must not be mixed: a reply to a "common sense" intervention by *Toxicology* journal editors. *Environmental Health* 2013;12:69. http://www.ehjournal.net/content/12/1/69; Bergman A et al. The impact of endocrine disruption: a consensus statement on the state of the science. *Environmental Health Perspectives* 2013;121:A104–A106; Gore AC et al. Policy decisions on endocrine disruptors should be based on science across disciplines: a response to Dietrich et al. *European Journal of Endocrinology* 2013;169:E1–E4.

64. Cressey D. Journal editors trade blows over toxicology: debate flares around European regulation of bisphenol A and other endocrine disrupters. *Nature News* 2013 Sept. 20.

65. Teeguarden et al. Twenty-four hour human urine.

66. Smith OW, Smith GV. Use of diethylstilbestrol to prevent fetal loss from complications of late pregrancy. *New England Journal of Medicine* 1949;241:562–68.

67. Testai et al. A plea for risk assessment.

68. Ibid.; Lamb et al. Critical comments; Goodman et al. Weight-of-evidence evaluation.

69. Sharpe RM. Is it time to end concerns over the estrogenic effect of bisphenol A? *Toxicological Science* 2010;114:1–4.doi:10.1093/toxsci/kfp299; Butterworth T. The scientists, the scare, the 100-million dollar surge. *Forbes* 2014 Apr. 9. http://www.forbes.com

/sites/trevorbutterworth/2014/04/09/bpa-the-scientists-the-scare-the-100-million-dollar-surge/.

70. Wilcox A, Herbst A. http://www.ncbi.nlm.nih.gov/pubmed/?term=wilcox+aj%2C+herbst+diethylstibestrol.

71. Interview with Allen Wilcox, Oct. 20, 2014.

72. Joffe. What has happened to human fertility?, 301.

73. Interview with Richard Sharpe, Aug. 21, 2014.

74. Ibid.

75. Interview with Daniel Doerge, Jan. 2, 2015.

76. Ibid.

77. Interview with Richard Sharpe.

78. Interview with Daniel Doerge. I should mention that a number of the researchers I interviewed regarding endocrine disruption asked that certain comments about specific researchers or institutions not be quoted. This is an important reminder of how even the most independent-minded scientists have to get along in the very small world of their specialized research area.

## 6. DEADLY REMEDY: A MYSTERIOUS DISEASE, A MEDICINAL HERB, AND THE RECOGNITION OF A WORLDWIDE PUBLIC HEALTH THREAT

1. Vanherweghem JL et al. Rapidly progressive interstitial renal fibrosis in young women: association with slimming regimes including Chinese herbs. *Lancet* 1993;341:387–91.

2. Cosyns JP et al. Chinese herbs nephropathy: a clue to Balkan endemic nephropathy? *Kidney International* 1994;45:1680–88; van Ypersele de Strihou C, Vanherweghem JL. The tragic paradigm of Chinese herbs nephropathy. *Nephrolology Dialysis Transplantation* 1995; 10:157–60.

3. Cosyns et al. Chinese herbs nephropathy.

4. Jadoul M, de Plaen JF, Cosyns JP, van Ypersele de Strihou C. Adverse effects from traditional Chinese medicine. *Lancet* 1993;341:892–93.

5. Cosyns JP, Jadoul M, Squifflet JP, van Cangh PJ, van Ypersele de Strihou C. Urothelial malignancy in Chinese herbs nephropathy. *Lancet* 1994;344:188.

6. Nortier JL et al. Urothelial carcinoma associated with the use of Chinese herb (Aristolochia fangchi). *New England Journal of Medicine* 2000;342:1686–92.

7. van Ypersele de Strihou, Vanherweghem. The tragic paradigm of Chinese herbs nephropathy.

8. Scarborough J. Ancient medicinal use of Aristolochia: birthwort's tradition and toxicity. *Pharmacy in History* 2011;53:3–21; Grollman AP, Scarborough J, Jelaković B. Aristolochic acid nephropathy: an environmental and iatrogenic disease. *Advances in Molecular Toxicology* 2009;3, chap. 7:211–27.

9. Kluthe R, Vogt A, Batsford S. Double blind study of the influence of aristolochic acid. *Arzneimittel-Forschung* 1982;32:443–45.

10. Mengs U, Lang W, Poch J-A. The carcinogenic action of aristolochic acid in rats. *Archives of Toxicology* 1982;51:107–19.

11. Schmeiser HH, Schoepe KB, Wiessler M. DNA Adduct formation of aristolochic acid I and II in vitro and in vivo. *Carcinogenesis* 1988;9:297–303.

12. Schmieser HH, Bieler CA, Wiessler M, van Ypersele de Strihou C, Consyns JP. Detection of DNA adducts formed by aristolochic acid in renal tissue from patients with Chinese herbs nephropathy. *Cancer Research* 1996;56:2025–28.

13. Nortier et al. Urothelial carcinoma.

14. International Agency for Research on Cancer. *Some Traditional Herbal Medicines, Some Mycotoxins, Naphthalene and Styrene*. IARC Monographs on the Evaluation of Carcinogenic Risks to Humans, vol. 82. Lyon, France: 2002.

15. Marcus DM, Grollman AP. Botanical medicines—the need for new regulation. *New England Journal of Medicine* 2002;347:2073–76.

16. Marcus DM, Grollman AP. Ephedra-free is not danger-free. *Science* 2003;301:1669–71.

17. The lecture is now incorporated into the online edition of the leading textbook of pharmacology, Goodman and Gilman's *The Pharmacological Basis of Therapeutics*.

18. Hranjec T et al. Endemic nephropathy: The case for chronic poisoning by Aristolochia. *Croatian Medical Journal* 2005;46:116–25.

19. Čeović S, Miletić-Medved M. Epidemiological features of endemic nephropathy in the focal area of Brodska Posavina. In *Endemic Nephropathy in Croatia*, ed. Čorišćec D, Čeović S, Stavljenić-Rukavina A, 7–21. Zagreb, Croatia: Academic Croatica Scientarium Medicarum, 1996.

20. Ibid.

21. Markovic B. Balkan nephropathy and urothelial cancer (in French). *Journal d'urologie* (Paris) 1990;96;349–52.

22. World Health Organization. Memorandum: the endemic nephropathy of south-eastern Europe. *Bulletin of the World Health Organization* 1965;32:441–48.

23. There was another important bit of misleading evidence: namely, the observation that ochratoxin causes cancer in the kidney—but not the urothelium—in one strain of male mice—and in fact is the most potent nephrocarcinogen ever reported in this test species. Although widely cited, this observation is irrelevant to human exposure since different tissues are involved.

24. Ivić M. The problem of aetiology of endemic nephropathy. *Acta Facultatis Medicae Naissensis* 1969;1:29–38.

25. Grollman AP et al. Aristolochic acid and the etiology of endemic (Balkan) nephropathy. *PNAS* 2007;104:12129–34. The kidney Grollman retrieved was that of a 39-year-old aerobics instructor from Cranston, Rhode Island, who, according to an article in *Consumer Reports*, had been prescribed over half a dozen Chinese herbs by her acupuncturist for health conditions, including endometriosis. She had been on the herbs for more than two years. At least one of the products contained *Aristolochia* as an ingredient, even though the FDA had issued a nationwide safety warning regarding *Aristolochia* in 2001.

26. Hranjec T, Brzić I. Eighty years of agricultural evolution: farming in Slavonski Brod. Unpublished report, May 1, 2006.

27. Ibid.

28. Grollman et al. Aristolochic acid.

29. Grollman, Scarborough, Jelaković. Aristolochic acid nephropathy.

30. Holstein M, Sidransky D, Vogelstein B, Harris CC. p53 mutations in human cancers. *Science* 1991;253:49–53.

31. Moriya M et al. TP53 mutational signature of aristolochic acid. *International Journal of Cancer* 2011;129:1532–36.

32. International Agency for Research on Cancer. IARC TP53 database. http://p53.iarc.fr/RefsDBanalysis.aspx.

33. Grollman, Scarborough, Jelaković. Aristolochic acid nephropathy.

34. Hoang ML et al. Mutational spectrum of aristolochic acid exposure as revealed by whole-exome sequencing. *Science Translational Medicine* 2013;15:197 197ra102.

35. Lai MN, Wang SM, Chen PC, Chen YY, Wang JD. Population-based case-control study of Chinese herbal products containing aristolochic acid and urinary tract cancer risk. *Journal of the National Cancer Institute* 2010;102:179–86.

36. Chen CH et al. Aristolochic acid-associated urothelial carcinoma in Taiwan. *PNAS* 2012;109(21):8241–46. doi:10.1073/pnas.1119920109. Epub 2012 Apr. 9.

37. Ibid.

38. Laing C, Hamour S, Sheaff M, Miller R, Woolfson R. Chinese herbal uropathy and nephropathy. *Lancet* 2006;368:338.

39. Ibid.

40. Personal communication with Arthur Grollman, Oct. 30, 2015.

41. Totoki Y et al. Trans-ancestry mutational landscape of hepatocellular carcinoma genomes. *Nature Genetics* 2014;46:1267–73. doi:10.1038/ng.3126; Scelo G et al. Variation in genomic landscape of clear cell renal cell carcinoma across Europe. *Nature Communications* 2014;5. doi:10.1038/ncomms6135.

42. Cohen PA. Hazards of hindsight—monitoring the safety of nutritional supplements. *New England Journal of Medicine* 2014;370:1277–80.

43. Offit PA. *Do You Believe in Magic? The Sense and Nonsense of Alternative Medicine.* New York: HarperCollins, 2013.

44. Cohen. Hazards of hindsight.

45. Ibid.

46. Ibid.; Offit. *Do You Believe in Magic?*, 91.

47. Adulteration of supplements with unapproved, banned, or untested drugs is a major problem, documented in more than five hundred instances. The contaminants include stimulants, anabolic steroids, antidepressants, weight-loss medications, and Viagra analogues (Cohen. Hazards of hindsight). Both adulterants and legal ingredients present in supplements have been linked to a wide range of potential adverse reactions, from arrhythmias, cancer, and liver damage to heart attacks and strokes (ibid.).

48. Marcus DM, Grollman AP. The consequences of ineffective regulation of dietary supplements. *Archives of Internal Medicine* 2012;172:1035–36.

49. Ibid.

50. Cohen. Hazards of hindsight.

51. Acute hepatitis and liver failure following the use of a dietary supplement intended for weight loss or muscle building—May–October, 2013. *MMWR Morbidity and Mortality Weekly* 2013;62:817–19.

52. Cohen. Hazards of hindsight. Grollman explained something that was not mentioned in the news reports, or even in medical articles, discussing the OxyElitePro incident. For OxyElitePro to qualify as an herbal supplement, the manufacturer USPLabs added a natural ingredient, aegeline, derived from the bael fruit, which is popular in China and India. However, the concentration used in OxyElitePro was many times higher than in the bael fruit. In effect, aegeline was being used as a drug. Unbelievably, an earlier formulation of OxyElitePro and another product, Jack3d, that contained the stimulant DMAA were linked to one hundred cases of illness and six deaths. After destroying the stocks of these products, USPLabs reformulated OxyElitePro and rereleased it. A month later the first reports of liver toxicity turned up in Hawaii.

53. Navarro VJ et al. Liver injury from herbals and dietary supplements in the U.S. drug-induced liver injury network. *Hepatology* 2014;60:1399–1408.

54. Geller AI et al. Emergency department visits for adverse events related to dietary supplements. *New England Journal of Medicine* 2015;373:1531–40.

55. Offit. *Do You Believe in Magic?*; Singh S, Ernst E. *Trick or Treatment: The Undeniable Facts About Alternative Medicine*. New York: Norton, 2009.

56. Another argument used by supporters of dietary supplements is that there are well-documented cases in which medications approved by the FDA have been shown to cause harm. But this argument doesn't stand up since, first, in order to be approved, medications have to have some evidence of effectiveness, and, second, due to regulation, drugs that show adverse effects are removed from the shelves. In fact, this argument favors tighter oversight of supplements.

## 7. HPV, CANCER, AND BEYOND: THE ANATOMY OF A TRIUMPH

1. Kevles, DJ. Pursuing the unpopular: a history of courage, viruses, and cancer. In *Hidden Histories of Science*, ed. Silver RB. New York: New York Review of Books, 1996; Stebbing J, Bower M. Epstein-Barr virus in Burkitt's lymphoma: the missing link. *Lancet Oncology* 2009:430.

2. Coakley D. Denis Burkitt and his contribution to haematology/oncology. *British Journal of Haematology* 2006;135:17–25. My account of Burkitt's work and Harald zur Hausen's early work on Epstein-Barr virus is based on the primary literature by Burkitt, zur Hausen, and their colleagues. After this chapter was written, *The Cancer Virus: The Story of Epstein-Barr Virus*, by Dorothy H. Crawford, Alan Rickinson, and Ingolfur Johannessen, was published. The early chapters of that book give a detailed account of the seminal research on the first human cancer virus.

3. Burkitt D. A Sarcoma involving the jaws of African children. *British Journal of Surgery* 1958;46:218–23.

4. Burkitt D. Determining the climatic limitations of a children's cancer common in Africa. *BMJ* 1962;2:1019–23; Burkitt D. A "tumor safari" in East and Central Africa. *British Journal of Cancer* 1962;16:379–86.

5. Burkitt. Determining the climatic limitations.

6. In "A 'Tumor Safari,'" Burkitt credited his colleague J. N. P. Davies for this insight.

7. Smith O. Denis Parsons Burkitt CMG, MD, DSc, FRS, FRCS, FTCD (1911–93) Irish by birth, trinity by the grace of God. *British Journal of Haematolology* 2012;156:770–76. Epstein A, Burkitt D. Sir Anthony Epstein, CBE FRS in conversation with Dr. Denis Burkitt, CMG, FRS, Oxford, 20 March 1991. Royal College of Physicians and Oxford Brookes University Medical Services Video Archive MSVA 059, Oxford Brookes University, Oxford, UK.

8. Coakley. Denis Burkitt.

9. Epstein MA, Achong BG, Barr YM. Virus particles in cultured lymphocytes from Burkitt's lymphoma. *Lancet* 1964; Mar. 28:702–3. This highly cited paper, half of which is taken up by two electron micrographs, is less than two pages long.

10. DeThé G et al. Epidemiological evidence for causal relationship between Epstein-Barr virus and Burkitt's lymphoma from Ugandan prospective study. *Nature* 1978;274:756–61.

11. Molyneux EM et al. Burkitt's lymphoma. *Lancet* 2012;379:1234–44. Molyneux points out that the story of Burkitt's lymphoma includes a number of important firsts. "Burkitt's lymphoma has had an important role in the understanding of tumorigenesis. It was the first human tumour to be associated with a virus, one of the first tumours shown to have a chromosomal translocation that activates an oncogene, and the first lymphoma reported to be associated with HIV infection. Burkitt's lymphoma is the fastest growing human tumour, with a cell doubling time of 24–48 h, and was the first childhood tumour to respond to chemotherapy alone. It is the most common childhood cancer in areas where malaria is holoendemic—e.g., equatorial Africa, Brazil, and Papua New Guinea. The so-called Burkitt's lymphoma belt stretches across central Africa 15° either side of the equator where the climate is hot and wet (more than 50 cm annual rainfall). The epidemiological maps of malaria and Burkitt's lymphoma overlap."

12. Ibid.

13. Stebbing, Bower. M. Epstein-Barr virus in Burkitt's lymphoma; Harald zur Hausen, Nobel lecture.

14. W. Henle papers, National Library of Medicine.

15. Castellsagué X, Bosch FX, Muñoz N. Environmental cofactors in HPV carcinogenesis. *Virus Research* 2002;89:191–99.

16. Hulka BS. Risk factors for cervical cancer. *Journal of Chronic Disease* 1982;35:3–11.

17. Ibid.

18. Schiffman MH, Hildsheim A. Cervical cancer. In *Cancer Epidemiology and Prevention*, ed. Schottenfeld D, Fraumeni JF Jr., 1044–67. New York: Oxford University Press, 2006.

19. Ibid.

20. Rotkin ID. A comparison review of key epidemiological studies in cervical cancer related to current searches for transmissible agents. *Cancer Research* 1973;33:1353–67.

21. Zur Hausen H. Papillomaviruses in the causation of human cancers—a brief historical account. *Virology* 2009;384:260–65.

22. Ibid.; Franco EL, Schlecht NF, Saslow D. The epidemiology of cervical cancer. *Cancer Journal* 2003;9:348–359.

23. Zur Hausen H. On the case (interview). *Nature* 2012;488:S16.

24. Ibid.

25. Ibid.

26. Stebbing, Bower. M. Epstein-Barr virus in Burkitt's lymphoma.

27. Zur Hausen. On the case.

28. Zur Hausen H. Roots and perspectives of contemporary papillomavirus research. *Journal of Cancer Research and Clinical Oncology* 1996;122:3–13. Koutsky L. The epidemiology behind the HPV vaccine discovery. *Annals of Epidemiology* 2009;19:239–244.

29. Hulka. Risk factors for cervical cancer.

30. Zur Hausen. Roots and perspectives.

31. Zur Hausen H. Cervical carcinoma and human papillomavirus: on the road to preventing a major human cancer. *Journal of the National Cancer Institute* 2001;93: 252–253.

32. Schiffman M, Wentzensen N. Human papillomavirus infection and the multistage carcinogenesis of cervical cancer. *Cancer Epidemiology Biomarkers and Prevention* 2012;22:553–60.

33. Ibid.

34. Ibid.

35. Ho GYF, Bierman R, Beardsley L, Chang CJ, Burk RD. Natural history of cervicovaginal papillomavirus infection in young women. *New England Journal of Medicine* 1998;338:423–28.

36. Interview with Robert Burk. Burk pointed out that in the early days herpes virologists "basically populated the scientific network of HPV research." Herpes is a latent virus—once infected with herpes, always infected with herpes. "So they brought with them the collective consciousness of continual persistence." Burk himself had worked on hepatitis B virus before turning to HPV. "The hepatitis B virus actually gets cleared from the body and is gone."

37. de Sanjosé S et al. Worldwide prevalence and genotype distribution of cervical human papillomavirus DNA in women with normal cytology: a meta-analysis. *Lancet Infectious Disease* 2007;7:453–59; Bosch FX et al. Epidemiology and natural history of human papillomavirus infections and type-specific implications in cervical neoplasia. *Vaccine* 2008;26S:K1–K16.

38. Bosch et al. Epidemiology and natural history; Ho et al. Natural history.

39. Schiffman, Wentzensen. Human papillomavirus infection.

40. Bosch et al. Epidemiology and natural history.

41. Schiffman, Wentzensen. Human papillomavirus infection.

42. Interview with Burk.

43. Schiffman, Wentzensen. Human papillomavirus infection.

44. Muñoz, N. Human Papillomavirus and cancer: the epidemiological evidence. *Journal of Clinical Virology* 2000;19:1–5.

45. Ibid.; Wallboomers JMM et al. Human papillomavirus is a necessary cause of invasive cervical cancer worldwide. *Journal of Pathology* 1999;189:12–19.

46. Franco, Schlecht, Saslow. Epidemiology of cervical cancer. Although the IARC study had an important impact, providing strong evidence for a causative role of HPV in cervical cancer, the decision to retest only those samples that were negative for HPV was shocking to those who are methodologically inclined. If you retest the negatives, the results can only get better! According to Burk, his epidemiologist colleagues "went nuts, went ballistic because that was just the wrong way to do it."

47. Ibid.

48. Castellsagué, Bosch, Muñoz. Environmental cofactors.

49. Tommasino M. The human papillomavirus family and its role in carcinogenesis. *Seminars in Cancer Biology* 2014;26:13–21.

50. Franco, Schlecht, Saslow. Epidemiology of cervical cancer.

51. Ibid.

52. Schiffman, Wentzensen. Human papillomavirus infection.

53. Zur Hausen. Papillomaviruses.

54. Ibid.

55. Ibid.

56. Scudellari M. Sex, cancer, and a virus. *Nature* 2013;503:330–32.

57. Ibid.

58. O'Connor A. Throat cancer link to oral sex gains notice. *New York Times* 2013 June 3.

59. STATBITE. Number of HPV-associated cancer cases per year in the United States (2004–2008). *Journal of the National Cancer Institute* 2013;105:998.

60. Peto J, Gilham C, Fletcher O, Matthews FE. The cervical cancer epidemic that screening has prevented in the UK. *Lancet* 2014;364:249–56.

61. Pollack A. F.D.A. panel recommends replacement for the Pap test. *New York Times* 2014 Mar. 18.

62. Interview with Burk.

63. Koutsky. Epidemiology behind the HPV vaccine discovery; Moscicki AB. HPV vaccines: today and in the future. *Journal of Adolescent Health* 2008;43 (Suppl):S26–S40.

64. Koutsky. Epidemiology behind the HPV vaccine discovery; Moscicki. HPV vaccines.

65. CDC. *Teen Vaccination Coverage.* 2014. http://www.cdc.gov/vaccines/who /teens/vaccination-coverage.html.

66. Ibid.

67. Carroll A. Good talks need to combat HPV vaccine myth. *New York Times* 2015 Nov. 9.

68. National Cancer Institute. Gardasil 9 vaccine protects against additional HPV types.    http://www.cancer.gov/types/cervical/research/gardasil9-prevents-more-HPV-types; Guliano AR, Kreimer AR, de Sanjosé S. The beginning of the end: vaccine prevention of HPV-driven cancers. *Journal of the National Cancer Institute* 2015;107:djv128. doi:10.1093/jnci/djv128.

69. Tota JE, Chevarie-Davis M, Richardson LA, deVries M, Franco EL. Epidemiology and burden of HPV infection and related diseases: implications for prevention strategies. *Preventive Medicine* 2011;53:S12–S21.

70. Ibid.

71. Arbyn M et al. Worldwide burden of cervical cancer in 2008. *Annals of Oncology* 2011;22:2675–86.

72. de Sanjosé et al. Worldwide prevalence.

73. Schiffman M, Castle PE. The promise of global cervical-cancer prevention. *New England Journal of Medicine* 2005;353:2101–04.

74. Mills A. Health care systems in low- and middle-income countries. *New England Journal of Medicine* 2014;370:552–57.

75. Ibid.; Cohen SA. A long and winding road: getting the HPV vaccine to women in the developing world. *Guttmacher Policy Review* 2007;10:15–19; Bharadwaj M, Hussain S, Nasare V, Das BC. HPV and HPV vaccination: issues in developing countries. *Indian Journal of Medical Research* 2009;130:327–33; Agosti JM, Goldie SJ. Introducing HPV vaccine in developing countries—key challenges and issues. *New England Journal of Medicine* 2007;356:1908–10; Bello FA, Enabor OO, Adewole IF. Human papilloma virus vaccination for control of cervical cancer: a challenge for developing countries. *African Journal of Reproductive Health* 2011;15:25–30.

76. GAVI the Vaccine Alliance. *Human papillomavirus vaccine support.* http://www.gavi.org/support/nvs/human-papillomavirus-vaccine-support/.

77. Schiffman, Castle. Promise of global cervical-cancer prevention.

78. Agosti, Goldie. Introducing HPV vaccine in developing countries.

79. Interview with Burk.

80. Ibid.

81. Burk RD, Chen Z, van Doorslaer K. Human papillomaviruses: genetic basis of carcinogenicity. *Public Health Genomics* 2009;12:281–90.

82. Ong CK et al. Evolution of human papilloma virus type 18: an ancient phylogenetic root in Africa and intratype diversity reflect coevolution with human ethnic groups. *Journal of Virology* 1993;67:6424–31.

83. Ibid.

84. Ho L et al. The genetic drift of human papillomavirus type 16 is a means of reconstructing prehistoric viral spread and the movement of ancient populations. *Journal of Virology* 1993;67:6413–23.

85. Interview with Burk.

86. Burk, Chen, van Doorslaer. Human papillomaviruses

87. Lai TK, Spitz M, Schully SD, Khoury MJ. "Drivers" of translational cancer epidemiology in the 21st century: needs and opportunities. *Cancer Epidemiology Biomarkers Prevention* 2012;22:181–88.

88. Burkitt's career includes four remarkable achievements. Soon after arriving in Uganda in 1946, he investigated the occurrence of hydrocele—the collection of fluid in the scrotum, which he found occurred with a frequency of 30 percent in one area but at only 1 percent in another area. He proposed that the condition was caused by filariasis—a parasitic disease caused by threadlike worms that burrow through the skin and get into the bloodstream and certain tissues. This hypothesis was borne out by further research. Second was his mapping of Burkitt's lymphoma. Third was his contribution to the development of successful chemotherapy regimens to treat Burkitt's lymphoma. Finally, starting in the 1970s, he took up and promoted the idea that many of the chronic diseases common in developed societies but rare in Africa (such as colorectal cancer, diabetes, and diverticulitis) could be ascribed to the low level of dietary fiber in the typical Western diet.

89. Coakley. Denis Burkitt.

# CONCLUSION

1. Collins H. *Are We All Scientific Experts Now?* Malden, Mass.: Polity Press 2014.

2. Tsilidis KT, Papatheordorou SI, Evangelou E, Ioannidis JPA. Evaluation of excess statistical significance in meta-analyses of 98 biomarker associations with cancer risk. *Journal of the National Cancer Institute* 2012;104:1867–75.

3. Sharpe RM. Lessons learned from andrology: learning from experience—getting it wrong is alright. *Andrology* 2014;2:652–54.

4. Khoury MJ, Ioannidis JP. Big data meets public health. *Science* 2014;28;346:1054–55. doi:10.1126/science.aaa2709.

# GLOSSARY

**ADENOCARCINOMA** A malignant tumor formed from glandular structures in epithelial tissue. It is the predominant cell type in breast, pancreatic, prostate, and colorectal cancers. Adenocarcinoma of the cervix is the second most common type after squamous cell carcinoma.

**AFLATOXIN** Poisonous and cancer-causing chemicals that are produced by certain molds which grow in soil, decaying vegetation, hay, and grains. They are regularly found in improperly stored staple commodities such as cassava, chili peppers, corn, cotton seed, millet, peanuts, rice, sorghum, sunflower seeds, tree nuts, wheat, and a variety of spices.

**ALKYLPHENOLS** Class of organic compounds. Long-chain alkylphenols are used extensively as precursors to the detergents and are also used in making many industrial and consumer products. They have received attention for their weak endocrine effects.

**ANTIBODY** A protein produced by the immune system to identify and neutralize pathogens such as bacteria and viruses. The antibody recognizes a unique molecule of the harmful agent, called an antigen.

**ASSOCIATION** A correlation between an exposure, or a characteristic, and a disease. Association is a necessary condition for a causal relationship, but many phenomena are associated without one of them causing the other. Hence the dictum "association does not prove causation."

**ATRAZINE** A common herbicide used on important food crops such as corn, sorghum, and sugar cane.

**AVAILABILITY CASCADE** A self-reinforcing process of collective belief formation by which an expressed perception triggers a chain reaction that gives the perception of increasing plausibility through its rising availability in public discourse.

**AVAILABILITY HEURISTIC** A mental shortcut that relies on immediate examples that come to a given person's mind when evaluating a specific topic, concept, method, or decision.

**BAYES' THEOREM** A valuable tool for judging how a subjective degree of belief should rationally change to account for available evidence. Bayes' theorem describes the probability of an event, based on conditions that might be related to the event. For example, suppose one is interested in whether a woman has cancer, and knows that she is 65. If cancer is related to age, information about her age can be used to more accurately assess the probability of her having cancer using Bayes' theorem.

**BIAS** Deviation of results or inferences from the truth, or processes leading to such deviation. Any trend in the collection, analysis, interpretation, or review of data that can lead to conclusions that are systematically different from the truth.

**BISPHENOL A (BPA)** Compound used to line food containers and in the manufacture of polycarbamate plastics.

**CARCINOMA** A type of cancer that develops from epithelial cells, that is, in a tissue that lines the inner or outer surfaces of the body. These are the most common types of cancer.

**CASE-CONTROL STUDY** Type of study in which cases of a particular disease are identified and a comparison group without the disease (controls) is identified. Information on factors thought to play a role in the disease is obtained from both groups and compared. Case-control studies are particularly useful in studying uncommon diseases.

**CAUSALITY** Agency or efficacy that connects one process with another, where the first is understood to be partly responsible for the second.

**CAUSATION** A means of connecting an event or exposure with a resulting effect.

**COHORT STUDY** Study in which information relevant to the risk of developing disease is collected from members of a defined population, or "cohort." The cohort is then followed for a number of years, and cases (or deaths) of the disease of interest are identified. Factors associated with the development of disease can then be evaluated.

COMPLEMENTARY AND ALTERNATIVE MEDICINE (CAM): ALTERNATIVE MEDICINE is any practice that is put forward as having the healing effects of medicine but does not originate from evidence gathered using the scientific method, is not part of biomedicine, or is contradicted by scientific evidence or established science. COMPLEMENTARY MEDICINE is alternative medicine used together with conventional medical treatment, in a belief, not confirmed using the scientific method, that it "complements" (improves the efficacy of) the treatment.

CONFIDENCE INTERVAL A measure of the reliability of a risk estimate. A 95 percent confidence interval means that 95 times out of 100 the estimated risk will fall within the specified interval.

CONFOUNDING, CONFOUNDING FACTOR The distortion of an observed association between a factor of interest and a disease by a third factor that is associated with both the study factor and the disease.

CRITERIA OF JUDGMENT A set of considerations elaborated by the statistician Austin Bradford Hill relevant to judging whether an observed association is causal. These include the strength of the association, the consistency of the association observed in different studies, temporality (whether the exposure precedes the occurrence of disease), and biological plausibility.

CRYPTORCHIDISM (UNDESCENDED TESTES) The failure of one or both of the testicles to move down from the abdomen into the scrotum. It is the most common birth defect of the male genitalia.

CYTOLOGY The study of cells; more specifically, in the context of cervical cancer, the examination of cells obtained via Pap testing to identify cancerous changes.

DDT (DICHLORODIPHENYLTRICHLOROETHANE) An organochlorine compound widely used as an agricultural insecticide following World War II. DDT was banned in the United States for agricultural use starting in 1972.

DEMING The high rate of publication of results from observational studies that cannot be replicated. The term refers to Edwards Deming, an innovator in quality control in the automobile industry, who argued that (1) a system that is out of control is not the fault of the workers, it is the fault of the managers that designed and run the system; and (2) it is the responsibility of managers to fix the system.

DIETARY SUPPLEMENTS Dietary supplements include vitamins, minerals, herbals and botanicals, amino acids, enzymes, and many other products.

**DIETARY SUPPLEMENT AND HEALTH EDUCATION ACT (DSHEA)** A U.S. federal statute, passed in 1994, which defines vitamin, mineral, herbal, and other products as "dietary supplements." Dietary supplements are exempt from the rigorous standards that apply to drugs, and manufacturers are not required to provide evidence of safety or efficacy in order to market a product.

**DIETHYLSTILBESTROL (DES)** A synthetic, nonsteroidal estrogen that was administered to pregnant women in the middle of the twentieth century to prevent miscarriage.

**DIOXIN** The common name for the chemical 2,3,7,8-tetrachlorodibenzo-p-dioxin, or TCDD. The term "dioxins" refers to a group of dioxin-like chemical compounds that share similar chemical structures. Most dioxins are produced through burning and other industrial activities. They are highly toxic and persistent in the environment and accumulate exponentially as they move up the food chain.

**DNA ADDUCT** A piece of DNA covalently bonded to a (cancer-causing) chemical. This process could be the start of a cancerous cell, or carcinogenesis.

**DOSE-RESPONSE RELATIONSHIP** The change in risk of disease (response) as exposure to the factor of interest (dose) increases. The number of cigarettes smoked per day by smokers shows a classic dose-response relationship with their risk of lung cancer.

**EBOLA** A rare and deadly disease caused by infection with a strain of Ebola virus, first identified in 1976 in Central Africa. The Ebola epidemic in 2014 was the largest in history, affecting multiple countries in West Africa. The risk of an Ebola outbreak affecting large numbers of people in the United States is very low.

**ELECTROMAGNETIC FIELD (EMF)** A physical field produced by electrically charged objects. It affects the behavior of charged objects in the vicinity of the field. The electromagnetic field extends indefinitely throughout space and describes the electromagnetic interaction.

**ELECTROMAGNETIC SPECTRUM** The range of all possible electromagnetic radiation from gamma rays, with very high frequencies and energies, to extremely low-frequency fields from power lines and electric appliances that have very low energy levels.

**ENDOCRINE DISRUPTING CHEMICALS** Term used to identify chemicals in the environment that can interfere with normal hormonal pathways, including estrogen, testosterone, and thyroid hormones. However, the label is often used loosely based on limited studies that are often not applicable to real-world exposure and do not distinguish between irreversible effects and transient effects. The term often presupposes that which it aims to prove.

**ENDOCRINE DISRUPTION** Exposure to certain drugs or possibly to chemicals in the environment can disrupt the endocrine system by mimicking a natural hormone, by blocking the effects of a hormone from certain receptors, or by directly stimulating or inhibiting the endocrine system and causing overproduction or underproduction of hormones.

**ENVIRONMENT** Used in the health sciences to refer broadly to exposures other than genetic inheritance. Thus the term includes not just industrial pollution but other "external" exposures, including diet, smoking, microbes, drugs, etc.

**EPITHELIAL TISSUE** A sheet of cells that covers a body surface, such as the skin, or lines organs, such as the lungs and digestive tract.

**ESTRADIOL** More precisely, 17β-estradiol, a steroid and estrogen sex hormone, and the primary female sex hormone. It is named for and is important in the regulation of the estrous and menstrual female reproductive cycles.

**EXPOSURE** The condition of having contact with a physical or chemical agent in such a way that the contact can influence the development of disease.

**FALSE POSITIVE RESULT** A result, showing a positive association, that proves to be wrong when evaluated using better evidence.

**FERTILITY** The natural capability to produce offspring. As a measure, fertility rate is the number of offspring born per mating pair, individual, or population.

**FRACKING (HYDRAULIC FRACTURING)** The process of drilling and injecting fluid into the ground at a high pressure in order to fracture shale rocks to release natural gas inside.

**FREQUENCY (ELECTROMAGNETIC WAVES)** Number of oscillations per unit time, i.e., number of cycles per second (hertz).

**GENETIC MODIFICATION** Also called genetic engineering. The direct manipulation of an organism's genome using biotechnology. It is a set of technologies used to change the genetic makeup of cells, including the transfer of genes within and across species boundaries to produce improved or novel organisms.

**GENOME-WIDE ASSOCIATION STUDY (GWAS)** An approach that involves rapidly scanning markers across the complete sets of DNA, or genomes, of many people to find genetic variations associated with a particular disease.

**GENOMICS** A discipline in genetics that applies recombinant DNA, DNA sequencing methods, and bioinformatics to sequence, assemble, and analyze the function and structure of genomes (the complete set of DNA within a single cell of an organism).

**GLIOMA** Type of primary brain tumor, accounting for about one-third of all brain tumors. Gliomas originate in the glial cells, which surround and support neurons in the brain. Glioma is the most fatal type of brain tumor.

**GLYPHOSATE** A broad-spectrum systemic herbicide and an organophosphorus compound, used to kill weeds, especially annual broadleaf weeds and grasses that compete with crops.

**HAZARD** The potential of an exposure to cause harm and adverse effects.

**HAZARD IDENTIFICATION** Identification of a potential risk due to a particular compound or agent.

**HEAD AND NECK CANCER** Cancers that usually begin in the squamous cells that line the moist, mucosal surfaces inside the head and neck, including the mouth, pharynx, larynx, and esophagus.

**HELICOBACTER PYLORI** A bacterium found usually in the stomach that is also linked to the development of duodenal ulcers and stomach cancer.

**HERPES SIMPLEX VIRUS 2 (HSV-2)** Member of the herpesvirus family that infect humans. HSV-2 (which produces most genital herpes) is ubiquitous and contagious.

**HEURISTIC** Any approach to problem solving, learning, or discovery that employs a practical method not guaranteed to be optimal or perfect but sufficient for the immediate goals. Heuristics can be mental shortcuts that ease the cognitive load of making a decision. Examples of this method include using a rule of thumb, an educated guess, an intuitive judgment, stereotyping, profiling, or common sense.

**HORMONE** Any member of a class of signaling molecules produced by glands in multicellular organisms that are transported by the circulatory system to target distant organs to regulate physiology and behavior.

**HUMAN PAPILLOMAVIRUS (HPV)** A DNA virus from the papillomavirus family that is capable of infecting the skin and mucous membranes of humans.

**HYPOSPADIAS** A birth defect of the urethra in the male where the urinary opening is not at the usual location on the head of the penis. It is the second most common birth abnormality in boys, affecting approximately 1 of every 250.

**INCIDENCE RATE** The frequency of newly diagnosed cases of a disease within a period of time (usually one year). Cancer incidence is often reported in terms of the number of new cases per hundred thousand population.

**INFERENCE** Drawing conclusions about a population using data drawn from the population by means of sampling.

**IN SITU HYBRIDIZATION** A powerful technique that uses a labeled complementary DNA, RNA, or modified nucleic acids strand (i.e., probe) to localize a specific DNA or RNA sequence in a portion or section of tissue (in situ), providing insights into physiological processes and disease pathogenesis.

**INTERNATIONAL AGENCY FOR RESEARCH ON CANCER (IARC)** An arm of the World Health Organization, which conducts cancer research and publishes assessments of potential cancer causing substances.

**INTERNATIONAL COMMITTEE ON NON-IONIZING RADIATION PROTECTION (ICNIRP)** An independent organization that provides scientific advice and guidance on the health and environmental effects of non-ionizing radiation to protect people and the environment from detrimental non-ionizing radiation.

**INTERPHONE STUDY** A large international case-control study led by IARC to examine the association of mobile phone use and brain tumors.

**IONIZING RADIATION** Electromagnetic radiation with sufficient energies to dislodge electrons from an atom, thereby producing an ion pair. Ionizing radiation includes gamma rays, X-rays, and alpha-particles, which can damage DNA through ionization.

**ISOFLAVONE** A type of phytoestrogen, or plant hormone, that resembles human estrogen in chemical structure yet is weaker.

**MENINGIOMA** A diverse group of tumors arising from the meninges, the membranous layers surrounding the central nervous system. These tumors are usually benign; however, a small percentage are malignant.

**META-ANALYSIS** A technique used to combine the results of a number of small studies in order obtain a summary estimate (basically, a weighted average of the smaller studies), which, it is hoped, will better describe the association. Meta-analysis can be carried out using the data available from published papers, in contrast to pooled analyses, which involve reanalyzing the original data from different studies using a common approach.

**METABOLISM** The set of life-sustaining chemical transformations within the cells of living organisms. These enzyme-catalyzed reactions allow organisms to grow and reproduce, maintain their structures, and respond to their environments. The word metabolism can also refer to all chemical reactions that occur in living organisms, including digestion and the transport of substances into and between different cells.

**MICROWAVES** A form of electromagnetic radiation with wavelengths ranging from one meter to one millimeter; with frequencies between 300 MHz (100 cm) and 300 GHz (0.1 cm). The prefix "micro" indicates that microwaves have "small" wavelengths compared to waves used in typical radio broadcasting.

**MUTATION** A permanent alteration of the nucleotide sequence of the genome of an organism, virus, or extrachromosomal DNA or other genetic elements.

**NEPHROTOXIN** A toxic agent or substance that inhibits, damages, or destroys the cells and/or tissues of the kidneys.

**NONMONOTONIC DOSE-RESPONSE (NMDR)** Controversial concept according to which exposure to a compound at a low level can have a greater effect than exposure at a higher level. This contrasts with the widely accepted notion of a monotonic dose-response relationship in which greater exposure is associated with larger effects. NMDR is currently being evaluated by the U.S. Environmental Protection Agency.

**OBSERVATIONAL STUDY** A study in which subjects are enrolled and provide information about their health history and exposures and personal habits, which is then correlated with information about the development of a disease(s) of interest. This type of study is contrasted with an experimental study, such as a randomized controlled clinical trial, in which the researcher allocates participants to either the intervention group or the control (placebo) group.

**OCHRATOXIN** A group of fungal toxins produced by some *Aspergillus* species and some *Penicillium* species. Ochratoxin A is the most prevalent and relevant fungal toxin of this group.

**ODDS RATIO** The measure of association obtained from a case-control study, compares the "odds" of exposure to the factor of interest among cases to the odds of exposure among the controls.

**ONCOGENE** A gene that in certain circumstances can transform a cell into a tumor cell.

**ORAL CANCER/ORAL CAVITY CANCER** Can develop in any part of the oral cavity (the mouth and lips) or the oropharynx (the part of the throat at the back of the mouth).

**ORGANOCHLORINE COMPOUNDS** A wide range of chemicals that contain carbon, chlorine, and sometimes several other elements. A range of organochlorine compounds have been produced, including many herbicides, insecticides, fungicides, as well as industrial chemicals such as polychlorinated biphenyls (PCBs).

**OROPHARYNX** Part of the throat at the back of the mouth.

**PAP TEST (PAPANICOLAOU TEST)** A method of cervical screening, known earlier as Pap smear, cervical smear, or smear test, used to detect potentially precancerous and cancerous processes in the cervix (opening of the uterus or womb).

**PHARMACOKINETIC MODEL** A mathematical modeling technique for predicting the absorption, distribution, metabolism, and excretion (ADME) of synthetic or natural chemical substances in humans and other animal species. PBPK modeling is used in pharmaceutical research and drug development, and in health risk assessment for cosmetics or general chemicals.

**PHYTOESTROGENS** Plant-derived xenoestrogens not generated within the endocrine system but consumed by eating phytoestrogenic plants. Also called "dietary estrogens," they are a diverse group of naturally occurring nonsteroidal plant compounds that, because of their structural similarity with estradiol (17-β-estradiol), have the ability to cause estrogenic or/and antiestrogenic effects by sitting in and blocking receptor sites against estrogen.

**POLYCHLORINATED BIPHENYLS (PCBs)** A group of man-made compounds that were widely used in the past, mainly in electrical equipment, but were banned at the end of the 1970s in many countries because of environmental concerns.

**POLYMERASE CHAIN REACTION (PCR)** A technology in molecular biology used to amplify a single copy or a few copies of a piece of DNA across several orders of magnitude, generating thousands to millions of copies of a particular DNA sequence.

**PRECAUTIONARY PRINCIPLE** Approach to risk management that states that if an action or policy has a suspected risk of causing harm to the public or to the environment, in the absence of scientific consensus that the action or policy is not harmful, the burden of proof that it is *not* harmful falls on those taking an action.

**PROSPECTIVE STUDY** See cohort study.

**RADIATION** Energy emitted in the form of waves or particles by radioactive atoms as a result of radioactive decay.

**RADIOFREQUENCY (RF) WAVES** Another name for radio waves. This form of electromagnetic energy consists of waves of electric and magnetic energy moving together (radiating) through space. RF wave frequencies lie in the range extending from around 3 kHz to 300 GHz, which include those frequencies used for communications or radar signals.

**RECALL BIAS** Differential reporting of exposure information by cases and controls in a case-control study. May be due to cases' desire to find an explanation for their diagnosis or to the effects of disease on their recall of past events.

**RELATIVE RISK** The ratio of the risk of disease or death among the exposed to the risk among the unexposed.

**RENAL CORTEX** The outer portion of the kidney where ultrafiltration occurs.

**RENAL PELVIS** Part of the kidney that serves as a funnel for urine flowing into the ureter.

**RISK** The probability that an event will occur, e.g., the probability that an individual will become ill or die within a stated period of time or by a certain age.

**RISK ASSESSMENT** The determination of quantitative or qualitative estimate of risk related to a concrete situation and a recognized threat (also called hazard).

**RISK FACTOR** A personal characteristic or exposure that in an epidemiologic study is associated with the occurrence of disease. Often the term is used to imply a causal relationship, when this is not appropriate.

**SPECIFIC ABSORPTION RATE (SAR)** Rate at which RF energy is absorbed by human tissues.

**SELECTION BIAS** Error due to systematic differences in characteristics between those who take part in a study and those who do not. Selection bias can invalidate conclusions and generalizations that might otherwise be drawn from a study.

**SEROLOGY** The scientific study of serum and other bodily fluids. In practice, the term usually refers to the diagnostic identification of antibodies in the serum.

**SINGLE NUCLEOTIDE POLYMORPHISM (SNP)** A variation in a single nucleotide that may occur at some specific position in the genome, where each variation is present to some appreciable degree within a population (e.g., greater than 1%).

**SQUAMOUS CELL CARCINOMA** A cancer of one type of epithelial cell, the squamous cell. Squamous cells are the main part of the skin but also occur in the lining of the digestive tract, lungs, and other areas of the body, and squamous cell carcinoma occurs in diverse tissues, including the lips, mouth, esophagus, urinary bladder, prostate, lung, vagina, and cervix, among others.

**STATISTICAL POWER** The ability of a study to detect a statistically significant association between an exposure and a disease of interest. Statistical power depends on the size of the study and how well the factors and the disease condition have been measured (i.e., on the quality of the data).

**STATISTICAL SIGNIFICANCE** A measure of whether a particular result is unlikely to be due to chance. If the 95 percent confidence interval associated with a relative risk (or odds ratio) does not include 1.0, the result is conventionally judged to be statistically significant.

**TESTICULAR DYSGENESIS SYNDROME (TDS)** A group of abnormalities of the male reproductive system including testicular cancer, impaired semen quality, undescended testis, and hypospadias.

**TRANSPLACENTAL CARCINOGENESIS** A series changes in the cells of a fetus due to in utero exposure to carcinogens that can result in the development of cancer.

**TUMOR SUPPRESSOR GENE** Gene that protects a cell from one step on the path to cancer. When this gene mutates to cause a loss or reduction in its function, the cell can progress to cancer, usually in combination with other genetic changes.

**UPPER UROTHELIAL CANCER, OR UPPER URINARY TRACT CANCER** Cancers of the upper urinary tract are relatively rare. In 2015 about 3,100 Americans will be diagnosed with this cancer. The most common of all upper urinary tract cancers are those found in the renal pelvis and renal calyces. Cancer in the ureters makes up about a quarter of all upper urinary tract cancers.

**UROTHELIAL CANCER** Cancer of the urinary system: predominantly those of the bladder, ureter, and urethra, but also less commonly in the kidney. These are transitional cell cancers and are distinct from renal cell cancers, which are the most common type of kidney cancer.

**WEIGHT-OF-THE-EVIDENCE ASSESSMENT** An approach used to integrate evidence from multiple lines of investigation in order to draw conclusions about a potential risk to a population.

# BIBLIOGRAPHY

Acute hepatitis and liver failure following the use of a dietary supplement intended for weight loss or muscle building—May–October. *MMWR Morbidity and Mortality Weekly* 2013;62:817–19.

Adair RK. Biophysical limits on athermal effects of RF and microwave radiation. *Bioelectromagnetics* 2003;24:39–48.

Agosti JM, Goldie SJ. Introducing HPV vaccine in developing countries—key challenges and issues. *New England Journal of Medicine* 2007;356:1908–10.

Ahlbom A, Feychting M. Mobile telephones and brain tumors (editorial). *BMJ* 2011;343. d6605. doi:10.1136/bmj.d6605.

Ahlbom A, Feychting M, Green A, Kheifets I, Savitz DA, Swerdlow AJ, ICNIRP (International Commission for Non-Ionizing Radiation Protection) Standing Committee on Epidemiology. Epidemiologic evidence on mobile phones and tumor risk: a review. *Epidemiology* 2009;20:639–52.

Ahlbom A, Green A, Kheifets L, Savitz D, Swerdlow A. Epidemiology of health effects of radiofrequency exposure. *Environmental Health Perspectives* 2004;112:1741–54.

Alberts B, Kirschner MW, Tilghman S, Varmus H. Rescuing US biomedical research from its systemic flaws. *Proceedings of the National Academy of Sciences U.S.A.* 2014;111:5773–77.

American Institute for Cancer Research. New survey: U.S. beliefs about cancer risk put fear before facts." 2015 Feb. 4.

Ames B, Gold LS. Paraselsus to parascience: the environment cancer distraction. *Mutation Research* 2000;447:3–13.

Arbyn M, Castellsagué X, de Sanjosé S, Bruni L, Saraiya M, Bray F, Ferlay J. Worldwide burden of cervical cancer in 2008. *Annals of Oncology* 2011;22:2675–86.

Associated Press. Cellphones a "possible" carcinogen—like coffee." *Seattle Times* 2011 June 1.

Atkinson RL, Macdonald I. White hat bias: the need for authors to have the spin stop with them (editorial). *International Journal of Obesity* 2010;34:83.

Bello FA, Enabor OO, Adewole IF. Human papilloma virus vaccination for control of cervical cancer: a challenge for developing countries. *African Journal of Reproductive Health* 2011;15:25–30.

Bergman A, Anderson A-M, Becher G, et al. Science and policy on endocrine disrupters must not be mixed: a reply to a "common sense" intervention by toxicology journal editors. *Environmental Health* 2013;12:69. http://www.ehjournal.net /content/12/1/69.

Bergman A., Heindel JJ, Jobling S, Kidd KA, Zoeller RT, eds. *Endocrine Disrupting Chemicals 2012: The State of the Science*. Geneva: World Health Organization and United Nations Environment Programme, 2013. http://www.who.int/ceh /publications/endocrine/en/.

Bergman A, Heindel JJ, Kasten T, Kidd KA, Jobling S, Neira M, Zoeller RT, Becher G, Bjerregaard P, Bornman R, Brandt I, Kortenkamp A, Muir D, Drisse M-NB, Ochieng R, Skakkebaek NE, Byléhn AS, Iguchi T, Toppari J, Woodruff TJ. The impact of endocrine disruption: a consensus statement on the state of the science. *Environmental Health Perspectives* 2013;121:A104–A106.

Bharadwaj M, Hussain S, Nasare V, Das BC. HPV and HPV vaccination: issues in developing countries. *Indian Journal of Medical Research* 2009;130:327–33.

Bhopal R. Seven mistakes and potential solutions in epidemiology, including a call for a world council of epidemiology and causality. *Emerging Themes in Epidemiology* 2009;6:6. doi:10.1186/1742-7622-6-6.

Bienkowsky B. BPA may prompt more fat deposition in the human body. *Scientific American*, May 29, 2015.

Birnbaum LS, Bucher JR, Collman GW, Zeldin DC, Johnson AF, Schug TT, Heindel JJ. Consortium-Based Science: The NIEHS's multipronged, collaborative approach to assessing the health effects of bisphenol A. *Environmental Health Perspectives* 2012;120:1640–44.

Boffetta P, McLaughlin JK, La Vecchia C, Tarone RE, Lipworth L, Blot WJ. False positive results in cancer epidemiology: a plea for epidemiologic modesty. *Journal of the National Cancer Institute* 2008;100:988–95.

Boisen KA, Main KM, Rajpert-de-Meyts E, Skakkebaek NE. Are male reproductive disorders a common entity? *Annals of the New York Academy of Sciences* 2001;948:90–99.

Bosch FX, Burchell AN, Schiffman M, Giuliano AR, de Sanjosé S, Bruni L, Tortolero-Luna G, Kjaer SK, Muñoz N. Epidemiology and natural history of human papillomavirus infections and type-specific implications in cervical neoplasia. *Vaccine* 2008;26S:K1–K16.

Bracken MB. *Risk, Chance, and Causation: Investigating the Origins and Treatment of Disease*. New Haven, Conn.: Yale University Press, 2013.

Bretveld RI, Thomas CMG, Scheepers PTJ, Zielhuis GA, Roeleveld N. Pesticide exposure: the hormonal function of the female reproductive system disrupted? *Reproductive Biology and Endocrinology* 2006;4:30. doi:10.1186/1477-7827-4-30.

Burk RD, Chen Z, van Doorslaer K. Human papillomaviruses: genetic basis of carcinogenicity. *Public Health Genomics* 2009;12:281–90.

Burkitt D. Determining the climatic limitations of a children's cancer common in Africa. *British Medical Journal* 1962;2:1019–23.

——. A sarcoma involving the jaws of African children. *British Journal of Surgery* 1958;46:218–23.

——. A "tumor safari" in East and Central Africa. *British Journal of Cancer* 1962;16:379–86.

Butterworth T. The scientists, the scare, the 100-million dollar surge. *Forbes* 2014 April 9. http://www.forbes.com/sites/trevorbutterworth/2014/04/09/bpa-the-scientists-the-scare-the-100-million-dollar-surge/.

Calafat AM, Koch HM, Swan SH, Hauser R, Goldman LR, Lanphear BP, Longnecker MP, Rudel RA, Teitelbaum SL, Whyatt RM, Wolff MS. Misuse of blood serum to assess exposure to bisphenol A and phthalates. *Breast Cancer Research* 2013;15:403.

Carlsen E, Giwercman A, Keiding N, Skakkebaek NE. Evidence for decreasing quality of semen during past 50 years. *BMJ* 1992;305:609–13.

Carroll A. Good talks need to combat HPV vaccine myth. *New York Times* 2015 Nov. 9.

Castellsagué X, Bosch FX, Muñoz N. Environmental cofactors in HPV carcinogenesis. *Virus Research* 2002;89:191–99.

Centers for Disease Control and Prevention. *CDC Estimates of Foodborne Illness in the United States 2014.* http://www.cdc.gov/foodborneburden/.

Čeović S, Miletić-Medved M. Epidemiological features of endemic nephropathy in the focal area of Brodska Posavina. In *Endemic Nephropathy in Croatia.* Edited by Čorišćec D, Čeović S, Stavljenić-Rukavina A, 7–21. Zagreb, Croatia: Academic Croatica Scientarium Medicarum, 1996.

Chang K. Debate continues on hazards of electromagnetic waves. *New York Times* 2014 July 7.

Chen CH, Dickman KG, Moriya M, et al. Aristolochic acid-associated urothelial carcinoma in Taiwan. *PNAS* 2012 109(21):8241–46. doi:10.1073/pnas.1119920109. Epub 2012 Apr 9.

Coakley D. Denis Burkitt and his contribution to haematology/oncology. *British Journal of Haematology* 2006;135:17–25.

Cohen PA. Hazards of hindsight—Monitoring the safety of nutritional supplements. *New England Journal of Medicine* 2014;370:1277–80.

Cohn BA, La Merrill M, Krigbaum NY, Yeh G, Park JS, Zimmerman L, Cirillo PM. DDT exposure in utero and breast cancer. *Journal of Endocrinology and Metabolism* 2015;100:2865–72.

Colborn T, Dumanoski D, Myers JP. *Our Stolen Future: Are We Threatening Our Fertility, Intelligence, and Survival? A Scientific Detective Story.* New York, NY: Plume, 1997.

Collins H. *Are We All Scientific Experts Now?* Malden, Mass.: Polity Press, 2014.

Cope MB, Allison DB. White hat bias: examples of its presence in obesity research and a call for renewed commitment to faithfulness in research reporting. *International Journal of Obesity* 2010;34:84–88.

Cosyns JP, Jadoul M, Squifflet JP, et al. Chinese herbs nephropathy: a clue to Balkan endemic nephropathy? *Kidney International* 1994;45:1680–88.

Cosyns JP, Jadoul M, Squifflet JP, van Cangh PJ, van Ypersele de Strihou C. Urothelial malignancy in Chinese herbs nephropathy. *Lancet* 1994;344:188.

Crawford DH, Rickinson A, Johannessen I. *The Cancer Virus: The Story of Epstein-Barr Virus*. New York: Oxford University Press, 2014.

Cressey D. Journal editors trade blows over toxicology: debate flares around European regulation of bisphenol A and other endocrine disrupters. *Nature News* 2013 Sept. 20.

Darwin C. *The Origin of Species*. Middlesex, UK: Penguin Books, 1970.

Davis D. Brain cancer and cell phones: the jury is still out. *Huffington Post* 2009 Dec. 7.

——. Cell phones and brain cancer: the real story. *Huffington Post* 2010 May 22.

——. *Disconnect: The Truth About Cell Phone Radiation, What the Industry Has Done to Hide It, and How to Protect Your Family*. New York: Dutton, 2010.

Davis DL, Bradlow HL, Wolff M, Woodruff T, Hoel DG, Anton-Culver H. Medical hypothesis: xenoestrogens as preventable causes of breast cancer. *Environmental Health Perspectives* 1993;101:372–77.

Dawkins R. *The Selfish Gene*. Oxford: Oxford University Press, 1976.

Deltour I, Auvinen A, Feychting M, Johansen C, Klaeboe L, Sankila R, Schüz J. Mobile phone use and incidence of glioma in the Nordic countries 1979–2008: consistency check. *Epidemiology* 2012;23:301–7.

Deltour I, Johansen C, Auvinen A, Feychting M, Klaeboe L, Schüz J. Time trends in brain tumor incidence rates in Denmark, Finland, Norway, and Sweden, 1974–2003. *Journal of the National Cancer Institute* 2009;101:1721–24.

DeThé G, Geser A, Day NE, Tukei PM, Williams EH, Beri DP, Smith PG, Dean AG, Bornkamm GW, Feorino P, Henle W. Epidemiological evidence for causal relationship between Epstein-Barr virus and Burkitt's lymphoma from Ugandan prospective study. *Nature* 1978;274:756–61.

De Vocht F, Burstyn I, Cherrie JW. Time trends (1998–2007) in brain cancer incidence rates in relation to mobile phone use in England. *Bioelectromagnetics* 2011;32:334–39.

Dietrich D, von Aulock S, Marquardt HWJ, Blaauboer BJ, Dekant W, Kehrer J, Hengstler JG, Collier AC, Gori GB, Pelkonen O, Lang F, Nijkamp FP, Stemmer K, Li A, Savolainen K, Hayes AW, Gooderham N, Harvey A. Open letter to the European Commission: scientifically unfounded precaution drives European Commission's recommendation on EDC reduction, while defying common sense, well-established science, and risk assessment principles. *Food Chemistry and Toxicology* 2013;62:A1–A4.

Dodds EC, Lawson W. Synthetic oestrogenic agents without the phenanthrene nucleus. *Nature* 1936;137:996–97.

Doerge DR, Twaddle NC, Woodling KA, Fisher JW. Pharmacokinetics of bisphenol A in neonatal and adult rhesus monkeys. *Toxicology and Applied Pharmacology* 2010 Oct 1;248:1–11. doi:10.1016/j.taap.2010.07.009. Epub 2010 Jul 23.

Dyson F. How to dispel your illusions, review of Daniel Kahneman, *Thinking, Fast and Slow*. *New York Review of Books* 2011 Dec. 22.

Elswick BA, Welsh F, Janzen DB. Effect of different sampling designs on outcome of endocrine disruptor studies. *Reproductive Toxicology* 2000;14:359–67.

Epstein A. Burkitt D. Sir Anthony Epstein, CBE FRS in conversation with Dr. Denis Burkitt, CMG, FRS, Oxford, 20 March 1991. Royal College of Physicians and Oxford Brookes University Medical Services Video Archive MSVA 059. Oxford Brookes University, Oxford, UK.

Epstein MA, Achong BG, Barr YJ. Virus particles in cultured lymphocytes from Burkitt's Lymphoma. *Lancet* 1964 Mar. 28: 702–3.

Engel SM, Wolff MS. Causal inference considerations for endocrine disruptor research in children's health. *Annual Review of Public Health* 2013;34:139–58.

Fairchild AL, Bayer R. Smoke and fire over e-cigarettes. *Science* 2015;347:375–76.

Feynman R. Cargo cult science: some remarks on science, pseudoscience, and learning how to not fool yourself. Commencement address, California Institute of Technology, 1974. http://calteches.library.caltech.edu/51/2/CargoCult.htm.

Fisch H. Declining worldwide sperm counts: disproving a myth. *Urology Clinics of North America* 2008;35:137–46.

Fisch H, Hyun G, Hensle TW. Rising hypospadias rates: disproving a myth. *Journal of Pediatric Urology* 2010;6:37–39.

Fisher JW, Twaddle NC, Vanlandingham M, Doerge DR. Pharmacokinetic modeling: prediction and evaluation of route dependent dosimetry of bisphenol A in monkeys with extrapolation to humans. *Toxicology and Applied Pharmacology* 2011 Nov 15;257(1):122–36. doi:10.1016/j.taap.2011.08.026. Epub 2011 Sep 2.

Franco EL, Schlecht NF, Saslow D. The epidemiology of cervical cancer. *Cancer Journal* 2003;9:348–59.

Freedman DH. Lies, damned lies, and medical science. *Atlantic* 2010 Nov. 20.

Frei P, Poulsen AH, Johansen C, Olsen JH, Steding-Jessen M, Schüz J. Use of mobile phones and brain tumors: update of Danish cohort study. *BMJ* 2011;343:d6387.

Geller AI, Shehab N, Weidle NJ, Lovegrove MC, Wolpert BJ, Timbo BB, Mozersky RP, Budnitz DS. Emergency department visits for adverse events related to dietary supplements. *New England Journal of Medicine* 2015;373:1531–40.

Goldberg P. Peers puzzled by Herberman's stance on cell phone while believers rally. *Cancer Letter* 2008;34, Aug. 1.

Goodman JE, Witorsch RJ, McConnell EE, Sipes IG, Slayton TM, Yu CJ, Franz AM, Rhomberg LR. Weight-of-evidence evaluation of reproductive and developmental effects of low doses of bisphenol A. *Critical Reviews in Toxicology* 2009;39(1):1–75. doi:10.3109/10408440903279946.

Gore AC, Bathazart J, Bikle D, Carpenter DO, Crews D, Czernichow P, Diamanti-Kandarakis E, Dores RM, Grattan D, Hof PR, Hollenberg AN, Lange C, Lee AV, Levine JE, Millar RP, Nelson RJ, Porta M, Poth M, Power DM, Prins GS, Ridgway EC, Rissman EF, Romijn JA, Sawchenko PE, Sly PD, Söder O, Taylor HS, Tena-Sempere M, Vaudry H, Wallen K, Wang Z, Wartofsky L, Watson CS. Policy decisions on endocrine disruptors should be based on science across disciplines: a response to Dietrich et al. *European Journal of Endocrinology* 2013;169:E1–E4.

Grollman AP, Scarborough J, Jelaković B. Aristolochic acid nephropathy: an environmental and iatrogenic disease. *Advances in Molecular Toxicology* 2009;3:211–27.

Grollman AP, Shibutani S, Moriya M, et al. Aristolochic acid and the etiology of endemic (Balkan) nephropathy. *PNAS* 2007;104:12129–34.

Guliano AR, Kreimer AR, de Sanjosé S. The beginning of the end: vaccine prevention of HPV-driven cancers. *Journal of the National Cancer Institute* 2015;107:djv128. doi:10.1093/jnci/djv128.

Gupta N, Stopfer M. Negative results need airing too. *Nature* 2011;470.

Hardell L, Carlberg M. Mobile phones, cordless phones and the risk for brain tumours. *International Journal of Oncology* 2009;35:5–17.

Hardell L, Carlberg M, Hansson MK. Pooled analysis of case-control studies on malignant brain tumours and use of mobile and cordless phones including living and deceased subjects. *International Journal of Oncology* 2011;38:1465–74.

Herbst AL, Ulfelder H, Poskanzer DC. Adenocarcinoma of the vagina: association of maternal stilbestrol therapy with tumor appearance in young women. *New England Journal of Medicine* 1971;284:878–81.

Hill AB. The environment and disease: association or causation? *Proceedings of the Royal Society of Medicine* 1965;58:295–300.

Ho GYF, Bierman R, Beardsley L, Chang CJ, Burk RD. Natural history of cervicovaginal papillomavirus infection in young women. *New England Journal of Medicine* 1998;338:423–28.

Ho L, Chan SY, Burk RD, et al. The genetic drift of human papillomavirus type 16 is a means of reconstructing prehistoric viral spread and the movement of ancient populations. *Journal of Virology* 1993;67:6413–23.

Hoang ML, Chen C-H, Sidorenko VS, et al. Mutational spectrum of aristolochic acid exposure as revealed by whole-exome sequencing. *Science Translational Medicine* 2013;15:197ra102.

Holstein M, Sidransky D, Vogelstein B, Harris CC. p53 mutations in human cancers. *Science* 1991;253:49–53.

Horton R. What is medicine's 5 sigma? *Lancet* 2015;385:1380.

Hranjec T, Kovac, A, Kos J, Mao W, Chen JJ, Grollman AP, Jelaković B. Endemic nephropathy: the case for chronic poisoning by aristolochia. *Croatian Medical Journal* 2005;46:116–25.

Hranjec T, Brzić I. Eighty years of agricultural evolution: farming in Slavonski Brod. Unpublished report, May 1, 2006, 33 pp.

Hulka BS. Risk factors for cervical cancer. *Journal of Chronic Disease* 1982;35:3–11.

Inskip PD, Hoover RN, Devesa SS. Brain cancer incidence trends in relation to cellular telephone use in the United States. *Neuro-Oncology* 2010;12:1147–51.

International Agency for Research on Cancer. *IARC Monographs on the Evaluation of Carcinogenic Risks to Humans.* Preamble. http://monographs.iarc.fr/ENG /Preamble/CurrentPreamble.pdf

International Agency for Research on Cancer. *IARC Monographs on the Evaluation of Carcinogenic Risks to Humans. Some Traditional Herbal Medicines, Some Mycotoxins, Naphthalene and Styrene.* 2002;82.

——. IARC TP53 database. http://p53.iarc.fr/RefsDBanalysis.aspx.

INTERPHONE Study Group. Brain tumours risk in relation to mobile telephone use: results of the INTERPHONE international case-control study. *International Journal of Epidemiology* 2010;39:675–94.

Ioannidis JPA. Contradicted and initially stronger effects in highly cited clinical research. *JAMA* 2005;294:218–28.

——. How to make more published research true. *PLoS Medicine* 2014;11(10):e1001747.

——. Why most research findings are false. *PLoS Medicine* 2005;2:e124. doi:10.1371/journal.pmed.0020124.

Ivić M. The problem of aetiology of endemic nephropathy. *Acta Facultatis Medicae Naissensis* 1970;1:29–38.

Jadoul M, de Plaen JF, Cosyns JP, van Ypersele de Strihou C. Adverse effects from traditional Chinese medicine. *Lancet* 1993;341:892–93.

Joffe M. Are problems with male reproductive health caused by endocrine disruption? *Occupational and Environmental Medicine* 2001;58:281–88.

——. Myths about endocrine disruption and the male reproductive system should not be propagated. *Human Reproduction* 2002;17:520–23.

——. Semen quality analysis and the idea of normal fertility. *Asian Journal of Andrology* 2010;12:79–82.

——. What has happened to human fertility? *Human Reproduction* 2010;25:295–307.

Joffe M, Holmes J, Jensen TK, Keiding N, Best N. Time trends in biological fertility in Western Europe. *American Journal of Epidemiology* 2013;178:722–30.

Jordan VC. Avoiding the bad and enhancing the good of soy supplements in breast cancer (editorial). *Journal of the National Cancer Institute* 2014;106:dju233.

Kabat G. After 40 years of research, what do we know about preventing breast cancer. *Forbes* 2013 Feb. 24.

——. Behind the World Health Organization's "cancerous" pronouncement on cell phones. *Forbes* 2011 Aug. 23.

——. The crisis of peer review. *Forbes* 2015 Nov. 23.

——. Having it both ways on what causes cancer: IARC's flawed paradigm. *Forbes* 2015 Nov. 19.

——. How activism distorts the assessment of health risks. *Forbes* 2012 Nov. 20.

——. *Hyping Health Risks: Environmental Hazards in Everyday Life and the Science of Epidemiology.* New York: Columbia University Press, 2008.

——. Making room for the unseen in tackling complex problems. *Forbes* 2013 Jan. 17.

Kahneman, D. *Thinking Fast and Slow.* New York: Farrar, Straus, and Giroux, 2011.

Kahneman D, Tversky A. Judgment under uncertainty: heuristics and biases. *Science* 1974;185:1124–31.

Kamrin MA. The "low dose" hypothesis: validity and implications for human risk. *International Journal of Toxicology* 2007;26:13–23.

Kevles DJ. Pursuing the unpopular: a history of courage, viruses, and cancer. In *Hidden Histories of Science*, ed. Silver RB. New York: New York Review of Books, 1996.

Khoury MJ, Ioannidis JP. Big data meets public health. *Science* 2014;346:1054–55.

Khurana VG, Teo C, Kundi M, Hardell L, Carlberg M. Cell phones and brain tumors: a review including the long-term epidemiologic data. *Surgical Neurology* 2009;72:205–14.

Kluthe R, Vogt A, Batsford S. Double blind study of the influence of aristolochic acid. *Arzneimittel-Forschung* 1982;32:443–45.

Kolata G. Sperm counts: some experts see a fall, others poor data. *New York Times* 1996 Mar. 19.

Konkel L. Data stretching back to 1959 may explain link between environment and breast cancer. *Scientific American*. http://www.scientificamerican.com/article /data-stretching-back-to-1959-may-explain-link-between-environment-and -breast-cancer/.

Koutsky L. The epidemiology behind the HPV vaccine discovery. *Annals of Epidemiology* 2009;19:239–44.

Krimsky S. *Hormonal Chaos: The Scientific and Social Origins of the Environmental Endocrine Hypothesis*. Baltimore: Johns Hopkins University Press, 2000.

Kuller L. Circular epidemiology. *American Journal of Epidemiology* 1999;150:897–903.

Kuran T, Sunstein CR. Availability cascades and risk regulation. Working Paper Series. http://www.law.uchicago.edu/Lawecon/index.html and at the Public Law and Legal Theory Working Paper Series, http://www.law.uchicago.edu/academics /publiclaw/index.html, and The Social Science Research Network Electronic Paper Collection, http://ssrn.com/abstract_id=1019644.

Kwon MS, Vorobyev V, Kännälä S, Laine M, Rinne JO, Toivonen T, Johansson J, Teräs M, Lindhom J, Alanko T, Hämäläinen J. GSM mobile phone radiation suppresses brain glucose metabolism. *Journal of Cerebral Blood Flow & Metabolism* 2011;31:2293–2301.

Lagorio S, Röösli M. Mobile phone use and risk of intracranial tumors: a consistency analysis. *Bioelectromagnetics* 2014;35:79–90.

Lai MN, Wang SM, Chen PC, Chen YY, Wang JD. Population-based case-control study of Chinese herbal products containing aristolochic acid and urinary tract cancer risk. *Journal of the National Cancer Institute* 2010;102:179–86.

Lai TK, Spitz M, Schully SD, Khoury MJ. "Drivers" of translational cancer epidemiology in the 21st century: needs and opportunities. *Cancer Epidemiology Biomarkers Prevention* 2012;22:181–88.

Laing C, Hamour S, Sheaff M, Miller R, Woolfson R. Chinese herbal uropathy and nephropathy. *Lancet* 2006;368:338.

Lamb JC IV, Boffetta P, Foster WG, Goodman JE, Hentz KL, Rhomberg LR, Staveley J, Swaen G, Van Der Kraak G, Williams AL. Critical comments on the WHO-UNEP State of the Science of Endocrine Disrupting Chemicals—2012. *Regulatory Toxicology and Pharmacology* 2014;69:22–40.

Landis SC, Amara SG, Asadullah K, Austin CP, Blumenstein R, Bradley EW, Crystal RG, Darnell RB, Ferrante RJ, Fillit H, Finkelstein R, Fisher M, Gendelman HE, Golub RM, Goudreau JL, Gross RA, Gubitz AK, Hesterlee SE, Howells DW, Huguenard J, Kelner K, Koroshetz W, Krainc D, Lazic SE, Levine MS, Macleod MR, McCall JM,

Moxley RT III, Narasimhan K, Noble LJ, Perrin S, PorterJD, Steward O, Unger E, Utz U, Silberberg SD. A call for transparent reporting to optimize the predictive value of preclinical research. *Nature* 2012;490:187–91.

Latour B. *We Never Have Been Modern*, trans. Catherine Porter. Cambridge, Mass.: Harvard University Press, 1993.

Linet MS, Inskip PD. Cellular (mobile) telephone use and cancer risk. *Reviews on Environmental Health* 2010;25:51–55.

Little MP, Rajaraman P, Curtis RE, Devesa SS, Inskip PD, Check DP, Linet MS. Mobile phone use and glioma risk: comparison of epidemiological study results with incidence trends in the United States. *BMJ* 2012;344:e1147. doi:10.1136/bmj.e1147.

Longnecker MP, Bellinger DC, Crews D, Eskenazi B, Silbergeld EK, Woodruff TJ, Susser ES. An approach to assessment of endocrine disruption in the National Children's Study. *Environmental Health Perspectives* 2003;111:1691–97.

Longnecker MP, Rogan WJ, Lucier G. The human health effects of DDT (dichlorodiphenyltrichloroethane) and PCBs (polychlorinated biphenyls) and an overview of organochlorines in public health. *Annual Review of Public Health* 1997;18:211–44.

Maharaj SV, Orem WH, Tatu CA, Lerch HE III, Szilagyi DN. Organic compounds in water extracts of coal: link to Balkan endemic nephropathy. *Environmental Geochemistry and Health* 2014;36:1–17.

Mangel M, Samaniego F. Abraham Wald's work on aircraft survivability. *Journal of the American Statistical Association* 1984,79:259–67.

Marcus DM, Grollman AP. Botanical medicines—the need for new regulation. *New England Journal of Medicine* 2002;347:2073–76.

——. The consequences of ineffective regulation of dietary supplements. *Archives of Internal Medicine* 2012;172:1035–36.

——. Ephedra-free is not danger-free. *Science* 2003;301:1669–71.

Markovic B. Balkan nephropathy and urothelial cancer (in French). *Journal d'urologie* (Paris) 1990;96:349–52.

McLachlan JA, Newbold RR, Burow ME, Li SF. From malformations to molecular mechanisms in the male: three decades of research on endocrine disrupters. *APMIS* 2001;109:263–272.

McLaughlin JK, Tarone RE. False positives in cancer epidemiology. *Cancer Epidemiology Biomarkers and Prevention* 2013;22:11–15.

Mengs U, Lang W, Poch J-A. The carcinogenic action of aristolochic acid in rats. *Archives of Toxicology* 1982;51:107–19.

Mills A. Health care systems in low- and middle-income countries. *New England Journal of Medicine* 2014;370:552–57.

Mnookin S. *The Panic Virus: The True Story Behind the Vaccine-Autism Controversy.* New York: Simon and Schuster, 2012.

Mooney C, Kirshenbaum G. *Unscientific America: How Scientific Illiteracy Threatens Our Future.* New York: Basic Books, 2009.

Molyneux EM, Rochford R, Griffen B, Newton R, Jackson G, Menon G, Harrison GJ, Israels T, Bailey S. Burkitt's lymphoma. *Lancet* 2012;379:1234–44.

Morabia A. *Enigmas of Health and Disease: How Epidemiology Helps Unravel Scientific Mysteries*. New York: Columbia University Press, 2014.

Moriya M, Slade N, Brdar B, et al. TP53 mutational signature of aristolochic acid. *International Journal of Cancer* 2011;129:1532–36.

Moscicki AB. HPV Vaccines: today and in the future. *Journal of Adolescent Health* 2008;43(Suppl):S26–S40.

Moulder JE, Foster KR, Erdreich LS, McNamee JP. Mobile phones, mobile phone base stations and cancer: a review. *International Journal of Radiation Biology* 2005;81:189–203.

Mukherjee S. Do cellphones cause brain cancer? *New York Times* magazine 2011 April 13.

Muñoz N. Human papillomavirus and cancer: the epidemiological evidence. *Journal of Clinical Virology* 2000;19:1–5.

Myung SK, Ju W, McDonnell DD, Lee YJ, Kazinets G, Cheng CT, Moskowitz JM. Mobile phone use and risk of tumors: a meta-analysis. *Journal of Clinical Oncology* 2009;27:5565–72. Epub 2009 Oct 13.

Nagel SC, vom Saal FS, Thayer KA, Dhar MG, Boechler M, Welshons WV. Relative binding affinity-serum modified access (rba-sma) assay predicts the relative in vivo bioactivity of the xenoestrogens bisphenol A and octylphenol. *Environmental Health Perspectives* 1997;105:70–76.

National Research Council. *Review of the Environmental Protection Agency's State-of-the-Science Evaluation of Nonmonotonic Dose-Response Relationships as They Apply to Endocrine Disrupters*. Washington, D.C.: National Academy of Sciences, 2014.

Navarro VJ, Barnhart H, Bonkovsky HL, et al. Liver injury from herbals and dietary supplements in the U.S.—drug-induced liver injury network. *Hepatology* 2014;60:1399–408.

Nohynek G, Borgert CJ, Dietrich D, Rozman KK. Endocrine disruption: fact or urban legend? *Toxicology Letters* 2013;223:295–305.

Nortier JL, Martinez MC, Schmeiser HH, et al. Urothelial carcinoma associated with the use of Chinese herb (*Aristolochia fangchi*). *New England Journal of Medicine* 2000;342:1686–92.

Nyhan B. To get more out of science, show the rejected research. *New York Times* 2014 Sept. 18.

O'Connor, A. Throat cancer link to oral sex gains notice. *New York Times* 2013 June 3.

Offit P. *Autism's False Prophets. Bad Science, Risky Medicine, and the Search for a Cure*. New York: Columbia University Press, 2010.

——. *Do You Believe in Magic? The Sense and Nonsense of Alternative Medicine*. New York: Harper, 2013.

Ong CK, Chan SY, Campo MS, et al. Evolution of human papilloma virus type 18: an ancient phylogenetic root in Africa and intratype diversity reflect coevolution with human ethnic groups. *Journal of Virology* 1993;67:6424–31.

Owens JW, Chaney JG. Weighing the results of differing "low dose" studies of the mouse prostate by Nagel, Cagen, and Ashby: quantification of experimental power and statistical results. *Regulatory Toxicology and Pharmacology* 2005;43:194–202.

Park R. *Voodoo Science: The Road from Foolishness to Fraud.* New York: Oxford University Press, 2000.

Park RL. Cellular telephones and cancer: how should science respond? *Journal of the National Cancer Institute* 2001;93:166–67.

Patel CJ, Cullen MR, Ioannidis JPA, Butte AJ. Systematic evaluation of environmental factors: persistent pollutants and nutrients correlated with serum lipids. *International Journal of Epidemiology* 2012;41:828–43.

Paulozzi LJ. International trends in rates of hypospadias and cryptorchidism. *Environmental Health Perspectives* 1999;107:297–302.

Peto J, Gilham C, Fletcher O, Matthews FE. The cervical cancer epidemic that screening has prevented in the UK. *Lancet* 2014;364:249–56.

Phillips CV, Goodman KJ. The missed lessons of Sir Austin Bradford Hill. *Epidemiologic Perspectives and Innovations.* 2004;1:3.

Platt JR. Strong inference. *Science* 1964;146:347–53.

Plummer B. The bacon freak-out: why the WHO's cancer warnings cause so much confusion. *Vox* 2015 Oct. 26.

Pollack A. F.D.A. Panel recommends replacement for the Pap test. *New York Times* 2014 March 18.

Quammen D. *The Chimp and the River: How AIDS Emerged from an African Forest.* New York: Norton, 2015.

———. *Spillover: Animal Infections and the Next Human Pandemic.* New York: Norton, 2013.

Rabins PV. *The Why of Things: Causality in Science, Medicine, and Life.* New York: Columbia University Press, 2013.

Repacholi MH, Lerchl A, Röösli M, et al. Systematic review of wireless phone use and brain cancer and other head tumors (review). *Bioelectromagnetics* 2012;33:187–206.

Rhodes R. *Deadly Feasts: Tracking the Secrets of a Terrifying New Plague.* New York: Simon and Schuster, 1997.

Rhomberg LR, Goodman JE. Low-dose effects and nonmonotonic dose-responses of endocrine disrupting chemicals: Has the case been made? *Regulatory Toxicology and Pharmacology* 2012;64:130–33.

Rhomberg LR, Goodman JE, Foster WG, Borgert CJ, van der Kraak C. A critique of the European Commission document "State of the Art Assessment of Endocrine Disrupters." *Critical Reviews in Toxicology* 2012 Jul;42(6):465–73. doi:10.3109/1040 8444.2012.690367.

Rogan WJ, Ragan NB. Evidence of effects of environmental chemicals on the endocrine system in children. *Pediatrics* 2003;112:247–52.

———. Some evidence of effects of environmental chemicals on the endocrine system in children. *Journal of Hygiene and Environmental Health* 2007;210:659–67.

Rothman KJ. Conflict of interest: the new McCarthyism in science. *Journal of the American Medical Association* 1993;269:2782–84.

———. Health effects of mobile telephones (editorial). *Epidemiology* 2009;20(5):653–55.

———. Six persistent research misconceptions. *Journal of General Internal Medicine* 2014;29:1060–64.

Rothman KJ, Greenland S. Causation and causal inference in epidemiology. *American Journal Public Health* 2005;95:S144–S150.

Rotkin ID. A comparison review of key epidemiological studies in cervical cancer related to current searches for transmissible agents. *Cancer Research* 1973;33:1353–67.

Safe SH. Clinical correlates of environmental endocrine disruptors. *Trends in Endocrinology and Metabolism* 2005;16:139–44.

——. Endocrine disruptors and human health—is there a problem? An Update. *Environmental Health Perspectives* 2000;108:487–93.

——. Is there an association between exposure to environmental estrogens and breast cancer? *Environmental Health Perspectives* 1997;105(Suppl. 3):675–78.

de Sanjosé S, Diaz M, Castellsagué X, Clifford G, Bruni L, Munoz N, Bosch FX. Worldwide prevalence and genotype distribution of cervical human papillomavirus DNA in women with normal cytology: meta-analysis. *Lancet Infectious Disease* 2007;7:453–59.

Saracci R, Samet J. Commentary: Call me on my mobile phone . . . or better not?—a look at the INTERPHONE study results. *International Journal of Epidemiology* 2010;39:695–98.

Satel SL. Will the F.D.A. kill off e-cigs? (op-ed). *New York Times* 2015 Jan. 18.

Savitz D. The etiology of epidemiologic perseveration: when enough is enough. *Epidemiology* 2010;21:281–83.

Savitz DA, Ahlbom A. Electromagnetic fields and radiofrequency radiation. In *Cancer Epidemiology and Prevention*. 3rd ed. Edited by Schottenfeld D, Fraumeni JF Jr. New York: Oxford University Press, 2006), 306–21.

Scarborough J. Ancient medicinal use of *Aristolochia*: birthwort's tradition and toxicity. *Pharmacy in History* 2011;53:3–21.

Scelo G, Riazalhosseini Y, Greger L, et al. Variation in genomic landscape of clear cell renal cell carcinoma across Europe. *Nature Communications* 2014;5(5135). doi:10.1038/ncomms6135.

Schiffman M, Castle PE. The promise of global cervical-cancer prevention. *New England Journal of Medicine* 2005;353:2101–4

Schiffman M, Hildsheim A. Cervical cancer. In *Cancer Epidemiology and Prevention*. Edited by Schottenfeld D, Fraumeni JF Jr., 1044–67. New York: Oxford University Press, 2006.

Schiffman M, Wentzensen N. Human papillomavirus infection and the multistage carcinogenesis of cervical cancer. *Cancer Epidemiology Biomarkers and Prevention* 2012;22:553–60.

Schmeiser HH, Bieler CA, Wiessler M, Van Ypersele de Strihou C, Consyns JP. Detection of DNA adducts formed by aristolochic acid in renal tissue from patients with Chinese Herbs nephropathy. *Cancer Research* 1996;56:2025–28.

Schmeiser HH, Schoepe KB, Wiessler M. DNA adduct formation of aristolochic acid I and II in vitro and in vivo. *Carcinogenesis* 1988;9:297–303.

Schoenfeld JD, Ioannidis JP. Is everything we eat associated with cancer? A systematic cookbook review. *American Journal of Clinical Nutrition* 2013;97:127–34.

Scientific Committee on Emerging and Newly Identified Health Risks (SCENIHR). *Potential Health Effects of Exposure to Electromagnetic Fields (EMF)* 2015:72–84.

Scudellari M. Sex, cancer, and a virus. *Nature* 2013;503:330–32.

Sharpe RM. Endocrine disruption and human health effects—a call to action. *Nature* 2011;7:633–34.

——. Environment, lifestyle and male infertility. *Baillière's Clinical Endocrinology and Metabolism* 2000;14:489–503.

——. Is it time to end concerns over the estrogenic effects of bisphenol A? *Toxicological Sciences* 2010;114:1–4. doi:10.1093/toxsci/kfp299.

——. Lessons learned in andrology: learning from experience—getting it wrong is alright. *Andrology* 2014;2:652–54. doi:10.1111/j.2047-2927.2014.00242.x.

——. Pathways of endocrine disruption during male sexual differentiation and masculinization. *Best Practice & Research: Clinical Endocrinology & Metabolism* 2006:20:91–110.114:1–4. doi:10.1093/toxsci/kfp299.

——. Sperm counts and fertility in men: a rocky road ahead. *EMBO Reports* (European Molecular Biology Organization) 2012 April. doi:10.1038/embor.2012.50.

Sharpe RM, Turner KJ, Sumpter JP. Endocrine disruptors and testis development (letter). *Environmental Health Perspectives* 1998;106:220–21.

Sheehan DM. Activity of environmentally relevant low doses of endocrine disruptors and the bisphenol A controversy: initial results confirmed. *Proceedings of the Society for Experimental Biology and Medicine* 2000;224:57–60.

Shermer M. *The Believing Brain: From Ghosts and Gods to Politics and Conspiracies—How We Construct Beliefs and Reinforce Them as Truths.* New York: Times Books, 2011.

Singh S, Ernst E. *Trick or Treatment: The Undeniable Facts About Alternative Medicine.* New York: Norton, 2009.

Skloot R. *The Immortal Life of Henrietta Lacks.* New York: Broadway Books, 2010.

Slovic P, ed. *The Perception of Risk.* London: Earthscan, 2000.

Smith O. Denis Parsons Burkitt CMG, MD, DSc, FRS, FRCS, FTCD (1911–93) Irish by birth, trinity by the grace of God. *British Journal of Haematolology* 2012;156:770–76.

Specter M. *Denialism: How Irrational Thinking Hinders Scientific Progress, Harms the Planet, and Threatens Our Lives.* New York: Penguin Press, 2009.

Stacy SL, Brink LL, Larkin JC, Sadovsky Y, Goldstein BD, Pitt BR, Talbot EO. Perinatal outcomes and unconventional natural gas operations in southwest Pennsylvania. *PLoS ONE* 2015 June 3.

STATBITE. Number of HPV-associated cancer cases per year in the United States (2004–2008). *Journal of the National Cancer Institute* 2013;105:998.

Stebbing J, Bower M. Epstein-Barr virus in Burkitt's lymphoma: the missing link. *Lancet Oncology* 2009;10:430.

Stevens WK. Pesticides may leave legacy of hormonal chaos. *New York Times* 1994 Aug. 23.

Sunstein CR. Beyond the precautionary principle. *John M. Olin Law & Economics Working Paper* no. 149 (2nd series), *Public Law and Legal Theory Working Paper* no. 38, 2003 January.

Taubes G. Diet advice that ignores hunger. *New York Times* 2015 Aug. 29.

——. Epidemiology faces its limits. *Science* 1995;269:164–69.

Teeguarden JG, Calafat AM, Ye X, Doerge DR, Churchwell MI, Gunawan R, Graham MK. Twenty-four-hour human urine and serum profile of bisphenol A during high dietary exposure. *Toxicological Sciences* 2011;123:48–57.

Teeguarden JG, Hanson-Drury S. A systematic review of bisphenol-A "low dose" studies in the context of human exposure: a case for establishing standards for reporting "low-dose" effects of chemicals. *Food Chemistry and Toxicology* 2013;62:935–48.

Teeguarden J, Hanson-Drury S, Fisher JW, Doerge DR. Are typical human serum BPA concentrations measurable and sufficient to be estrogenic in the general population? *Food Chemistry and Toxicology* 2013;62:949–63.

Testai E, Galli CL, Dekant W, Marinovich M, Piersma AH, Sharpe RM. A plea for risk assessment of endocrine disrupting chemicals. *Toxicology* 2013;314:51–59.

Thomas L. *Lives of a Cell: Notes of a Biology Watcher.* New York: Viking, 1974.

Tommasino M. The human papillomavirus family and its role in carcinogenesis. *Seminars in Cancer Biology* 2014;26:13–21.

Tota JE, Chevarie-Davis M, Richardson LA, deVries M, Franco EL. Epidemiology and burden of HPV infection and related diseases: implications for prevention strategies. *Preventive Medicine* 2011;53:S12–S21.

Totoki Y, Tatsuno K, Covington KR, et al. Trans-ancestry mutational landscape of hepatocellular carcinoma genomes. *Nature Genetics* 2014;46:1267–73. doi:10.1038/ng.3126.

Trinquart L, Johns DM, Galea S. Why do we think we know what we know? A metaknowledge analysis of the salt controversy. *International Journal of Epidemiology* 2016;45:251–60.

Tsilidis KT, Papatheodorou SI, Evangelou E, Ioannidis JAP. Evaluation of excess statistical significance in meta-analyses of 98 biomarker associations with cancer risk. *Journal of the National Cancer Institute* 2012;104:1867–75.

Tyl RW. Basic exploratory research versus guideline-compliant studies used for hazard evaluation and risk assessment: bisphenol A as a case study. *Environmental Health Perspectives* 2009;117:1644–51. doi:10.1289/chp.0900893.

——. The presence (or not) of effects from low oral doses of BPA. *Journal of Toxicological Science* 2009;34:587–88.

Vandenberg LN, Colborn T, Hayes B, Heindel JJ, Jacobs DR, Lee D-H, Myers JP, Shioda T, Soto AM, vom Saal FS, Welshons WV, Zoeller RT. Regulatory decisions on endocrine disrupting chemicals should be based on the principles of endocrinology. *Reproductive Toxicology* 2013;38:1–15. doi:10.1016/j.reprotox.2013.02.002.

Vandenberg LN, Maffini MV, Sonnenschein C, Rubin BS, Soto AM. Bisphenol-A and the great divide: a review of controversies in the field of endocrine disruption. *Endocrinology Reviews* 2009;30:75–95.

Vanherweghem JL, Depierreux M, Tielemans C, et al. Rapidly progressive interstitial renal fibrosis in young women: association with slimming regimes including Chinese herbs. *Lancet* 1993;341:387–91.

Vidaeff AC, Sever LE. In utero exposure to environmental estrogen and male reproductive health: a systematic review of biological and epidemiologic evidence. *Reproductive Toxicology* 2005;20:5–20.

de Villiers E-M. Cross-roads in the classification of papillomaviruses. *Virology* 2013;445:2–10.

Volkow ND, Tomasi D, Wang G-J, Vaska P, Fowler JS, Telang F, Alexoff D, Logan J, Wong C. Effects of cell phone radiofrequency signal exposure on brain glucose metabolism. *JAMA* 2011;305:808–13. doi:10.1001/jama.2011.186.

Vom Saal FS, Welshons WV. Evidence that bisphenol A (BPA) can be accurately measured without contamination in human serum and urine and that BPA causes numerous hazards from multiple routes of exposure. *Molecular and Cellular Endocrinology* 2014. http://dx.doi.org/10.1016/j.mce.2014.09.028.

Walboomers, JMM, Jacobs MV, Manos MM, Bosch FX, Kummer JA, Shah KV, Snijders PJF, Peto J, Meijer CLM, Muñoz N. Human papillomavirus is a necessary cause of invasive cervical cancer worldwide. *Journal of Pathology* 1999;189:12–19.

Watson CS. Progress in understanding endocrine disruption requires cross-disciplinary approaches and concepts. *Endocrine Disruptors* 2013:1:1, e26646.

Watson JD. *The Double Helix*. New York: Signet Books, 1968.

Wiedemann PM, Boerner FU, Repacholi MH. Do people understand IARC's 2B categorization of RF fields from cell phones? *Bioelectromagnetics* 2014;35:373–78.

Wilcox AJ, Bonde JPE. On environmental threats to male infertility. *Asian Journal of Andrology* 2013;15:199–200. doi:10.1038/aja.2012.153; published online 2013 Jan 21.

Wilson EO. *Sociobiology*. Cambridge, Mass.: Belknap Press of Harvard University Press, 1975.

World Health Organization. Memorandum: the endemic nephropathy of south-eastern Europe. *Bulletin of the World Health Organization* 1965;32:441–48.

Yong E. Replication studies: bad copy. *Nature* 2012 485:298–300.

Young SS, Karr A. Deming, data and observational studies: a process out of control and needing fixing. *Significance* 2011;8:116–20. Published online 2011 Aug. 25. doi:10.1111/j.1740–9713.2011.00506.x.

Zur Hausen H. Cervical carcinoma and human papillomavirus: on the road to preventing a major human cancer. *Journal of the National Cancer Institute* 2001;93:252–53.

——. On the case (interview). *Nature* 2012;488:S16.

——. Papillomaviruses in the causation of human cancers—a brief historical account. *Virology* 2009;384:260–65.

——. Roots and perspectives of contemporary papillomavirus research. *Journal of Cancer Research and Clinical Oncology* 1996;122:3–13.

# INDEX

Page numbers in *italics* refer to illustrations.

acrylamide, 114

Adair, Robert K., 78–79

advocacy, 44

aflatoxin, 133, 134

Africa, 144–48, *146*, 164, 203n11. *See also* Burkitt's lymphoma

alcohol consumption, 14, 16, 21, 38, 43, 179

Allison, David, 44

American Institute for Cancer Research (AICR), xvi

Angell, Marcia, 39

animal studies, 76–77, 78, 80–81, 94, 102, 105–6. *See also* wildlife

anogenital cancer, 158–59

*Are We All Scientific Experts Now?* (Collins), 175

*Aristolochia* (herb), 6–7, 118–19, 125–32, 134–41, 143, 200n25. *See also* aristolochic acid

aristolochic acid: aristolactam-DNA adducts, 128–29, 130, 131, 137–38, 139; aristolochic acid nephropathy, 6–7, 128–30, 180, 200n25; as carcinogen, 118–20, 131–34, 137–40 (*see also* urothelial cancer); first suggested as cause of Balkan nephropathy, 125–26; genetic susceptibility to, 134–36. See also *Aristolochia*; Balkan endemic nephropathy; Chinese herbs nephropathy

associations, 8–31; assessing causality, 6, 25–27; complexity of linkages, *16*, 16–17; concurrent exposures and variables (correlation globe), *17*, 17–18; confirming through repeated studies, 15–16; defined, 14; deming (data dredging) and, 20; determining through epidemiologic studies, 13–14; examples of accepted causal

associations (*continued*)
associations, 14–15; interpretation of, 36–37; level of statistical significance, 22; not proof of causation, 14, 37, 187n4; reasons for false findings, 22–25; reduced through meta-analysis, 22; strong vs. weak, 15–16; surfeit of, 19–22, *21*

availability cascades, 53–55, 84. *See also* information cascades

availability entrepreneurs, 54

Bacon, Francis, 30

Balkan endemic nephropathy: aristolochic acid linked to, 125–26; characteristics, 123–24; Chinese herbs nephropathy similar to, 117, 120, 123, 180; geographic distribution, 123–24, *123*; Grollman's and Jelaković's work on, 121, 122–23, 126–32, 137 (*see also* Grollman, Arthur); history of, 6–7, 123–26. See also *Aristolochia*; Chinese herbs nephropathy; urothelial cancer

bandwagon processes, 50, 112–13, 115. *See also* information cascades

Bayes, Thomas, 79

Benjamin, Sam, 122

Bernard, Hans-Ulrich, 171

Berry, Donald, 81–82

beta-carotene, 38

bias: attachment to a given position, 48–49; availability entrepreneurs and, 54; and the cell phone–cancer controversy, 68–75; cognitive shortcuts and biases, 51–53, 84; conflict of interest and, 46, 80–81; defined, 22–23; and false claims and misinformation, 177; and false findings, 22–23; ignoring contradictory studies, 49, 104–5; Ioannidis's work on, 24–25; magnifying glass/blinkering effect, 41–42, 188n13; against negative studies, 39, 41; positive findings given more attention/credence, xviii, 39–40, 48, 52, 71–72, 93–94; publication bias,

41; recall bias, in case-control studies, 64, 67–68, 70; research interpreted for partisan purposes, 82; "the science is the science" claim, 61; in study design, 26, 105–6; white hat bias (political correctness), 44

Big Data (data mining), 179

BioInitiative Report, 68, 70

"Biophysical Limits on Athermal Effects of RF and Microwave Radiation" (Adair), 78–79

bisphenol A. *See* BPA

blinding, 70–71

body weight, 11, 21, 43, 44, 179. *See also* body weight

bombers, Allied, 1–3

BPA (bisphenol A), 92, 101–7; adverse effects probably minimal, 9, 108; and the endocrine system, 91–92; exposure levels and dose-response, 103–4; human exposure levels and serum BPA levels, 106–8, 109; potency, 38–39, 109, 114; risk assessment, 10; routes of exposure, 104; scientific disagreement over, 102–8; studies and papers on, 8, 44, 102, 105–8; in thermal register receipt paper, 8–9

brain cancer, 61, 64, 65, 68, 76, *77*. *See also* cell phones and brain cancer

Brawley, Otis, xv

breast cancer: age at menarche and, 97 (*see also* endocrine disrupting chemicals); DES and, 98; dietary fat and, 21; environmental exposures and, 18–19, 43, 94–97; limited understanding of, 56; progress in treatment of, 28; statistics, 61

breastfeeding, 44

*British Medical Journal*, 85–86, 98–100, 106, 145–46

Brussels renal disease cluster, 116–18, 122–23, 131–32, 134–35, 140–41, 143, 180. See also *Aristolochia*; Balkan endemic nephropathy

Burk, Robert, 153, 160, 166–67, 169–70, 172, 204n36, 205n46

Burkitt, Denis Parsons, 144–46, 173, 180, 207n88

Burkitt's lymphoma, 144–48, 173, 180, 203n11, 207n88

Butterworth, Trevor, 196n47

CAM. *See* Complementary and Alternative Medicine

cancer: alcohol consumption and, 14, 16, 21; causal associations (examples), 14, 15–16; concern over environmental pollution as cause, 87–88 (*see also* BPA; DDT; endocrine disrupting chemicals); DES and, 86–87, 91–92, 97; dietary factors and, 20–22, 24; "environmental factors" defined, 87; increase in research and papers on, 19; infectious agents and, 24, 144–49, 180, 203n11 (*see also* cervical cancer; HPV); mechanisms of, 132–34, 135, 157; signature (fingerprint) mutations, 133; smoking and, 14, 15–16, 26. *See also* cell phones and brain cancer; electromagnetic fields; *and specific cancers, such as* urothelial cancer

carcinogens, 40–41. *See also* cancer; *and specific carcinogens*

Carlsen, E., 85. *See also* "Evidence for Decreasing Quality of Semen During the Past 50 Years"

Carson, Rachel, 87

case-control studies, 13; brain tumor studies, 64; cell phone RF exposure studies, 64–68; on HPV and cervical cancer, 156; recall bias, 64, 67–68, 70. *See also* epidemiologic studies

cash register receipts (thermal), 8–9

causality: assessing, 6, 25–27; association not proof of causation, 14, 37, 187n4; Hill "criteria of judgment," 25; multiple causes, 26

*Cell Phone Radiation: Science Review on Cancer Risks and Children's Health*, 68–69

cell phones and brain cancer, 59–84; biased reporting by activists, 68–74; causal association not supported, 66–67, 74–75, 76–77, 177; cell phone frequency range, 62, 78; COSMOS study, 193n55; Danish cohort study, 60, 61, 75; experimental (animal) studies, 76–77, 78, 80–81; Hardell studies, 67–68, 69–70, 75, 76; IARC report, 80–82, 193n53; ICNIRP report, 66–67, 68, 70, 72, 75; increased cell phone use, 60, 76, *77*; INTERPHONE study, 66, 68, 72, 74–75, 82, 192n35; meta-analyses, 70–71; public concern over, xv, 43, 59–60, 81, 83; "radiation," 61, 62; RF exposure levels, 62–63; study design and challenges, 63–66; Volkow study, 79–80. *See also* radiofrequency energy

*Cell Phones and Brain Tumors—15 Reasons for Concern: Science, Spin and the Truth Behind Interphone*, 68–69

Cellular Telecommunications Industry Association, 60

Centers for Disease Control and Prevention, 142, 161

Cervarix (vaccine), 161

cervical cancer, 149–50; adenocarcinoma, 149, 160; genetic basis of, 169; HPV and, 7, 29, 56, 151–67, 169–70; HSV-2 and, 49, 180; mechanism and timing of, 157, 169; Pap screening, 154, 160; prevalence and mortality rates, 159–60, 162–63, *163*; squamous cell carcinoma, 149; vaccines against, 7, 56, 161–62, 165–67; zur Hausen's work on, 149, 150–52, 180. *See also* HPV

Chamberlin, T. C., 30

chemical pollutants, *17*, 17–18. *See also* BPA; DDT; endocrine disrupting chemicals; pollutants, environmental

China, 138–40. *See also* Chinese
  traditional medicine
Chinese herbs nephropathy, 116–18, 120,
  122–23, 130–32, 134–35, 140–41, 143,
  180, 200n25. See also *Aristolochia*;
  Balkan endemic nephropathy
Chinese traditional medicine, 118–19, 122,
  136–40. See also *Aristolochia*; ephedra
cigarettes, electronic, 11
Cleave, Peter, 173
Cochrane, Sir Ralph, 1–2
cognitive biases and shortcuts, 36,
  51–53, 84
cohort studies, 13; brain tumor studies,
  64; cell phone-related studies, 60,
  61, 64–65, 75, 193n55; determining
  existence and measure of association
  through, 13–14; of girls, through
  menarche, 97; large studies, 19–20;
  many associations generated, 20,
  21; proliferation of, 19–20. *See also*
  epidemiologic studies
Cohort Study of Mobile Phone Use and
  Health (COSMOS), 193n55
Colborn, Theo, 88–89, 90
Collins, Harry, 175, 176
Complementary and Alternative
  Medicine (CAM), 122, 141
conflict of interest, 46, 80–81
consensus, in science, 49–50
Cope, Mark, 44
correlation globe, *17*, 17–18
COSMOS study, 193n55
Cosyns, Jean-Pierre, 117–18, 119
criteria of judgment, 25, 157. *See also*
  evidence
Croatia. *See* Balkan endemic nephropathy
cryptorchidism (undescended testes), 90,
  98, 101, 115

data: dredging, 20; mining, 179; missing
  data, 2–3. *See also* evidence
Davis, Devra, 71–72

DDE (dichlorodiphenyldichloroethylene),
  95–96. *See also* DDT
DDT (pesticide), 18–19, 43, 91–92, *92*,
  95–97
deming, 20
denialism, xvii
DES (estrogen diethylstilbestrol), 92; and
  cancer, 86–87, 97, 98; dosage, 98, 109,
  178; endocrine disruption hypothesis
  and, 91–92, 194n5; Wilcox's work on,
  111–12
de Villiers, Ethel-Michelle, 167–68
diet, xv, 20–22, 24, 179. *See also* body
  weight
dietary and herbal supplements, 7, 12,
  121–22, 141–43, 201n47, 202n52. See
  also *Aristolochia*; Chinese herbs
  nephropathy; Chinese traditional
  medicine
Dietary Supplement Health and
  Education Act (DSHEA), 121,
  141, 143
Dietrich, Daniel, 108–9
dioxins, 86, 114
*Disconnect: The Truth About Cell Phone
  Radiation, What the Industry Has
  Done to Hide It, and How to Protect
  Your Family* (Davis), 71–72
DMAA (dimethylamylamine), 142,
  202n52
DNA damage and cancer, 38, 121, 132–33;
  aristolochic acid and (aristolactam-
  DNA adducts), 119, 128–29, 131, 132–
  34, 137–40 (*see also* urothelial cancer);
  RF energy and, 72, 78
Dodds, Edward Charles, 102
Doerge, Daniel, 103, 113–14, 115
Doll, Sir Richard, 173
dose, 37–38
dose-response relationship, 103–4
Douglas, Michael, 159
Drug-Induced Liver Injury Network,
  142

DSHEA. *See* Dietary Supplement Health and Education Act

Dyson, Freeman, 1–3

Ebola, 8–10, 18

EBV. *See* Epstein-Barr virus

EC. *See* European Commission

electromagnetic fields (EMFs), 35, 61–62; BioInitiative Report and, 73; media reporting on, 35; public concern over, 11, 35, 43, 59, 60, 65–66; risk not supported by research, 35, 73. *See also* radiofrequency energy

electromagnetic spectrum, 61–62, 62

electronic cigarettes, 11

EMFs. *See* electromagnetic fields

endocrine disrupting chemicals, 85–115; concomitant factors ignored in research, 41, 105; controversy over, 6, 11, 71, 91, 102–15; critical overviews of the issue, 111–15; endocrine disruption hypothesis, 88–92, 96–97, 100–101, 104–5, 194nn9, 13, 197–98n61 (*see also* BPA; DDT); exposure levels (magnitude), 98, 103–4, 106–8, 109, 178; impact of disruption hypothesis on research, 112; McLachlan on, 194n5; mechanisms, 91–92, 92; negative studies, 111–12; potency, 38–39, 178; precautionary principle and, 109–10; public awareness/concern, 6, 10–11, 43; skepticism re, 94; studies and publications on, 88–90, 94–96, 102, 106–8, 111–12. *See also* BPA; DDT; DES; estrogen; male fertility

*Endocrine Disrupting Chemicals 2012: The State of the Science* (Bergman, et al.), 108, 197–98n61

endocrine system, 91

"environmental," as term, 87

environmental health: controversies over, 48–49 (*see also specific topics*); and male fertility, 85–86; rising concern over, 19, 86, 87. *See also* endocrine disrupting chemicals; pollutants, environmental; *and specific chemicals*

Environmental Protection Agency (EPA), 87, 108

"Environment and Disease, The: Association or Causation?" (Hill), 25

ephedra, 122, 142

epidemiologic studies, 12–19; critical assessment of, 5–6, 25–27; factors affecting interpretation of, 36–50 (*see also* interpretation and reporting of studies); media reporting on, 33, 34–35; meta-analysis, 22; poorly defined research, 56–57; Proteus phenomenon, 24; reasons for false findings, 22–25 (*see also* false findings); types of study design, 13 (*see also* case-control studies; cohort studies). *See also* associations; case-control studies; cohort studies; *and specific research areas*

epidemiology, 19, 28. *See also* epidemiologic studies

Epstein, Anthony, 147

Epstein-Barr virus (EBV), 147–49

estrogen: BPA as, 38–39 (*see also* BPA); Danish semen quality study and, 86; environmental estrogen hypothesis, 86, 88–89 (*see also* endocrine disrupting chemicals); estradiol, 92, 98, 102; function of, 91; oral contraceptives in sewage effluent, 114; timing of, 38. *See also* DES; endocrine disrupting chemicals; estrogenic chemicals; hormones: hormone therapy

estrogenic chemicals, 85–86, 88–89, 91–93, 92, 94, 102, 194n5. *See also* BPA; DDT; DES

European Commission (EC), 47, 108–9

European Food Safety Authority, 108, 109

evidence: critical assessment of, 25–27, 28, 48, 49; evaluating credibility, 23–24, 25; ignoring contradictory studies, 4, 49, 104–5

"Evidence for Decreasing Quality of
　Semen During the Past 50 Years"
　(Carlsen, et al.), 85–86, 88, 98–100
exclusion, need for, 31
experimental studies: animal endocrine
　disruption studies, 94; BPA and
　fetal development in mice, 102,
　105–6; chemical exposure timing and
　mammary tumors, 97; RF studies on
　animals, 76–77, 78, 80–81
exposure: causal factors difficult
　to determine with low-level
　environmental exposure, 92–94; DES
　vs. environmental contaminants,
　98, 109, 178; determining
　association between disease and,
　15–18; dose-response relationship,
　103–4; magnitude of, 18, 37–39, 98;
　measuring RF exposure, 64–65 (see
　also cell phones; radiofrequency
　energy); routes of exposure, 104;
　timing of, 38, 88–89. See also specific
　agents

failure, importance of, 178
false claims, 177. See also Wakefield,
　Andrew
false findings, 6; and availability errors,
　53; false positive results, 39, 69–70;
　and media reporting, 34; and need
　to view "latest study" in context, 55;
　reasons for, 22–25
false problems, 177
fat (dietary), 21
fat (weight). See body weight
FDA. See Food and Drug Administration
fear, xiii–xv, xv, 56–58. See also cognitive
　biases and shortcuts; public, the; and
　specific topics, such as cell phones
Federal Communications Commission
　(FCC), 63
fetal development, synthetic chemicals
　and, 86–87, 88–89, 98, 102, 104, 115,
　194n9. See also DES

findings: communication gulf in
　reporting to public, xvii; false positive
　results, 39, 69–70; Latour's "hybrid"
　concept and, 35; media reporting
　on, xiii–xv, 33, 34–35, 39–40; more
　attention to positive findings, xviii,
　39–40, 48, 52, 93–94; mystique of,
　176; "null" findings rarely published,
　41; refuted findings still cited, 24;
　translation of, 33. See also false
　findings
Fisch, Harry, 99–100
Fish, Stanley, 82
flu, seasonal, 10
Food and Drug Administration (FDA):
　aristolochic acid advisory, 120,
　200n25; BPA deemed safe, 108; drug
　approval by, 202n56; and herbal and
　dietary supplements, 121, 141–42;
　HPV-DNA test recommended over
　Pap screening, 160; HPV vaccines
　approved, 161
foodborne illnesses, 11
Franco, Eduardo, 156
fraudulent research, 11, 45, 185n3
funding: endocrine disruption hypothesis's
　impact on, 112–13; industry funding,
　46, 60, 73–74; for large cohort studies,
　19–20; narrowly-framed issues and, 5;
　public appeal vs. scientific merit, xvi,
　57; public fears useful to, xvi, 43–44

gamma rays, 59, 61–62, 62. See also
　radiation
Gardasil (vaccine), 161–62, 166
GAVI Alliance, 166
genetically modified foods. See GM
　(genetically modified) foods
genetics and genomics, 177, 179. See also
　HPV
genital warts, 149, 150–51
genome association studies, 135
GM (genetically modified) foods, 10,
　11, 177

Gore, Al, 89
Gore, Andrea, 109
government agencies, 43–44. *See also* regulatory action; regulatory community; *and specific agencies*
Great Lakes fish, 86
Greenland, Sander, 26–27, 47
Grollman, Arthur, 120–23, 139; and Balkan endemic nephropathy, 122–32, 180, 200n25; and the safety of supplements, 121–22, 142, 143, 202n52; and urothelial cancer, 130–40

Hardell, Lennart, 67–68, 69–70, 72, 75, 80–81
hazard: hazard identification, 110; vs. risk, 40–41, 48, 80, 110, 188n10
Henle, Werner and Gertrude, 148, 149
hepatitis B virus (HBV), 24, 56, 161, 204n36
herbal supplements. *See* dietary and herbal supplements
Herberman, Ronald, 68, 71
Herbst, Arthur, 87
Herpes simplex virus type 2 (HSV-2), 29, 49, 150–52, 180, 204n36
heuristics, 27, 52
Hill, Austin Bradford, 25
*Hormonal Chaos* (Krimsky), 90
hormones, 91; hormonal effects of estrogenic substances, 91–93, 92, 102 (*see also* BPA; DDT; DES); hormone therapy, 14, 16, 38, 49–50
HPV (human papillomavirus), 149–72; about, 149, 150–51, 153–54; and anogenital and oropharyngeal cancers, 158–59; and cervical cancer, 7, 24, 29, 56, 80, 151–67, 169–70 (*see also* cervical cancer); contributing factors to HPV research success, 172; difficult to study, 152–53; genome mapping, 170, 172; genotypes, 154, 157, 158, 160–62, 167–72, *168*; HPV DNA testing, 160–61; HPV story as model, 172–73; IARC and,

80, 156, 162, 170, 205n46; increased research on, 154–55; prevalence by region, 163–64, *164*; study methods, 205n46; vaccines against, 7, 56, 161–62, 165–67; worldwide variation and prehistoric viral spread, 171–72
*H. pylori*, 24, 29, 56
Hranjec, Tjaša, 129–30
HSV-2. *See* Herpes simplex virus type 2
Hulka, Barbara, 152
Human Genome Project, 179
human papillomavirus. *See* HPV
hybrids (objects of scientific study), 35, 110
hypospadias, 90, 98, 101
hypotheses: danger of believing, 46–47 (*see also* scientific method); formulating (framing), 28–29, 30–31, 113, 179–80; investment in, 4; multiple, 30; poorly specified, and unproductive research, 56–57

IARC. *See* International Agency for Research on Cancer
ICNIRP. *See* International Commission on Non-Ionizing Radiation Protection
illusion of validity, 1–2, 3, 4, 18
immune system, 184n4
India, 163
industry-funded studies, 46, 60, 73–74
information cascades, 6, 50, 53–55. *See also* availability cascades
inference, strong, 27
Institute of Electrical and Electronic Engineers, 63
International Agency for Research on Cancer (IARC), 80; and aristolochic acid, 120; cancer genetic sequences database, 133–34; and cell phone RF energy, 66, 74, 80–82, 193n53 (*see also* INTERPHONE study); DDT classified as possible carcinogen, 95; and hazard vs. risk, 40–41, 80, 188n10; and HPV-cervical cancer research, 80, 156, 162, 170, 205n46

International Commission on Non-Ionizing Radiation Protection (ICNIRP), 63, 66–67, 68, 70, 72, 75

*International Journal of Epidemiology*, 74, 192n35. *See also* INTERPHONE study

INTERPHONE study, 66, 68, 72, 74–75, 82, 192n35

interpretation and reporting of studies, 36–50; advocacy and political correctness, 44; biased interpretation, 82; causation assumed, 37; conflict of interest, 46, 80–81; consensus not always correct, 49–50; danger of believing one's hypothesis, 46–47; environmental health controversies, 48–49; exposure (dose), timing, and properties of agent, 37–39; false positive results and, 39, 69–70; hazard vs. risk, 40–41, 48, 80; magnifying glass/blinkering effect, 41–42, 188n13; and opposition to scientific consensus, 5; peer-review system, 44–45; positive findings given more attention/credence, xviii, 39–40, 48, 52, 71–72, 93–94; precautionary principle and, 47–48, 69, 72–73, 189n25; publication bias, 41; public fears useful to scientists, regulators, 43–44; public sensitized to certain threats, xiii–xv, 42–43; science that appeals to public vs. science focused on next research, 55–56. *See also specific topics and reports*

Ioannidis, John P., 21–25, 39, 53

Ivić, Milenko, 125–26

Jelaković, Bojan, 126–28, 130

Joffe, Michael, 99, 100–101, 112, 196n37

*Journal of the American Medical Association (JAMA)*, 79–80

*Journal of the National Cancer Institute (JNCI)*, 60, 95–96

journals, scientific/medical, 12, 34, 44–45, 46, 60. *See also specific publications*

Kahneman, Daniel, 1, 51–53, 84

Khurana, V. G., 70

kidney cancer, 118, 200n23. *See also* urothelial cancer

kidney disease/failure. *See* Balkan endemic nephropathy; Chinese herbs nephropathy

Kinzler, Ken, 135

Krimsky, Sheldon, 90, 194n13

Kupchan, Morris, 119

Kuran, Timur, 53–55, 84

*Lancet* (journal), 45, 89, 117, 185n3, 194n9

Lander, Eric, 179

Latour, Bruno, 35, 110

Lipshultz, Larry, 99

Li Shizen, 138

liver damage, 142, 202n52

longitudinal studies. *See* cohort studies

Longnecker, Matthew, 94

Love Canal incident, 53–54, 88

Madaus, Rolf, 119

magnifying glass effect, 41–42, 188n13

malaria, 146, 147–48, 203n11

male fertility, 85–86, 94, 98–101, 196n37. *See also* semen quality

male reproductive disorders, 85–86, 89, 98, 100–101. *See also* male fertility; semen quality; testicular dysgenesis syndrome

Marcus, Donald, 121–22, 142

Marshall, Barry, 29

McLachlan, John, 194n5

measles, outbreak, 11

media: and the cell phone–cancer controversy, 59–60, 192n35; EMF reporting, 35, 65; endocrine disrupters covered, 89–90; and funding, 43; more attention to positive findings, xviii, 39–40, 48, 93–94; newsworthiness vs. scientific value, xiii–xv, 57–58, 115; reporting of study results or risks

(generally), xiii–xv, 33, 34–35, 55; and the threshold of publication, 45
meta-analysis, 22. *See also specific topics and publications*
methodology, as issue, 103–4
microwaves, 38, 62, 63. *See also* electromagnetic fields
misinformation, 177
missing data, 2–3
Moskowitz, Joel, 70–71, 72
Moulder, John, 78
mutations, involved in cancer, 121, 133

Nagel, Susan C., 102, 105–6
nasopharyngeal carcinoma, 140–49
National Cancer Institute, 60, 87, 96, 119, 154, 155, 158, 170
National Health and Nutrition Examination Survey, 17–18, *17*
National Institute of Environmental Health Sciences, 96, 97, 103, 105, 121
National Institutes of Health (NIH), 43
"natural experiment," 124
natural history of cervical cancer, 153
*New England Journal of Medicine*, 87, 118, 120, 122–23
*New Yorker*, 41–42, *42*
nonmonotonic dose-response, 104
Nortier, J. L., 119

obesity. *See* body weight
observational studies. *See* epidemiologic studies
ochratoxin, 125, 200n23
odds ratio (defined), 13
oropharyngeal cancer, 158–59
*Our Stolen Future: Are We Threatening Our Fertility, Intelligence, and Survival? Scientific Detective Story* (Colborn), 89, 90
OxyElitePro, 142, 202n52

p53 gene, 133, 137. *See also* urothelial cancer

papillomavirus. *See* HPV
Pap (Papanicolaou) screening, 154, 160
Park, Robert L., 60
PCBs (polychlorinated biphenyls), 43, 86, 95
peer-review system, 44–45
pesticides and herbicides, 11, 86. *See also* DDT
Phalen, Robert, 43
Platt, John R., 30–31
plausibility, xiv
political correctness, 44
pollutants, environmental: atmospheric pollutants, 11, 38; chemical pollutants correlation globe, 17–18, *17*; endocrine disruption hypothesis, 88–91, 92, 96–97, 100–101, 194nn9, 13, 197–98n61; estrogenic chemicals, 85–86, 88–89, 91–92, 92, 94, 194n5; public concern over, 43, 86–88. *See also* BPA; DDT; endocrine disrupting chemicals
polychlorinated biphenyls. *See* PCBs
Popper, Karl, 30
precautionary principle, 47–48, 189n25; and the cell phone–cancer question, 69, 72–73, 81
preference falsification, 54
*Proceedings of the National Academy of Sciences USA*, 134, 137, 139
processed meats, 41
prospective studies. *See* cohort studies
public, the: and availability cascades, 53–55, 84; BPA fears, 102; and the cell phone–cancer question, xv, 43, 59–60, 81, 83 (*see also* cell phones and brain cancer); communication gulf in reporting findings to, xvii; denialism, xvii; EMFs feared, 11, 35, 43, 59, 60, 65–66; external causes preferred, 179; external or invisible threats of more concern to, 42–43; and false/exaggerated findings, xiii–xiv, 6; fears useful to scientists, regulators, 43–44, 113; health information desired,

public (*continued*)
55–56, 176; influence of, on science, 4–5, 31, 35, 93–94, 110; knowledge/awareness of real risks, xvi; potential associations perceived as causal, 18; precautionary principle and, 47–48; RF concerns, 6, 43, 59–61, 66; science that appeals to, vs. science focused on next research, 55–56, 113–14; social context of "scientific" messages, xvii, 83; trust in science declining, xvi, 175. *See also* society

publication bias, 41

publication of studies. *See* journals

*Public Library of Science Medicine* (journal), 22

radiation, 59, 97, 103, 133. *See also* electromagnetic fields; radiofrequency energy

radiofrequency energy (RF): causal association with brain cancer not supported, 76–78; cell phone frequency range, 62, 78; concern and controversy over, 6, 43, 59–61, 66; electromagnetic spectrum, 61–62, 62; experimental studies on animals, 76–77, 78, 80–81; exposure through cell phone use, 62–63 (*see also* cell phones and brain cancer); and glucose metabolism in the brain, 79–80; nature and potency of, 38; physiological effect unlikely, 78–79. *See also* cell phones and brain cancer

reasoning, 51–52

red meat, 21

regulatory action: dietary and herbal supplements and, 7, 121–22, 141–43; impetus for, xv, 33

regulatory community: BPA deemed safe, 108; cell phone SAR limits, 63; hazard confused with risk, 40–41, 48, 80; more attention to positive findings, xviii, 39–40, 48; public fears useful to, 43–44

relative risk (defined), 13

resource allocation, xv–xvi

Reynard, David, 59, 61, 83–84, 190n1

RF. *See* radiofrequency energy

Rigoni-Stern, Domenico Antonio, 149–50

risk evaluation: exposure (dose), timing, and properties of agent, 37–39; hazard vs. risk, 40–41, 48, 80, 188n10; magnifying glass/blinkering effect, 41–42, 188n13; public fears and, 43–44

risk management: cell phone–cancer question, 72–73, 81, 193n53; precautionary principle and, 47–48, 72–73, 81, 189n25

Rothman, Kenneth, 26–27, 46, 60

Rous, Peyton, 144, 150

Safe, Stephen, 94, 103

salt intake, 11, 49

SCENIHR, 77

Schiffman, Mark, 155

Schmeiser, Heinz, 119

Schoenfeld, J. D., 21

science: bad vs. good, 5; characteristics leading to progress, 28–29; defined, 27; framing scientific questions, 113, 178 (*see also* hypotheses); heuristics and, 27; model for, 180; promise of, 179; public trust in, xvi, 175; public's knowledge of, 27; simplification/distortion of, 176–77. *See also* scientific establishment; scientific method; scientists

*Science* (journal), 30

Scientific Committee on Emerging and Newly Identified Health Risks (SCENIHR), 77

scientific establishment: and Complementary and Alternative Medicine (CAM), 122; consensus not always correct, 49–50; overhaul needed, 115; overturning dogma/paradigms of, 29; Platt on, 30–31;

relationship between society and, xvii, 5, 32–34, 33, 175–76
scientific method, 4, 28–29, 30–31, 46–47. See also hypotheses
scientists, 49; acknowledging what is/is not known, 177; advocacy and political correctness, 44; attachment to a given position, 48–49; as availability entrepreneurs, 54–55; and the cell phone–cancer controversy, 68–70; conflict of interest, 46, 80–81; consensus not always correct, 49–50; danger of believing one's hypothesis, 46–47; disagreements among, 11, 49, 71, 102–15, 176; and peer review, 44–45; public fears useful to, 43–44
semen quality, 85–86, 88, 94, 98–100, 106, 196n37
Sharpe, Richard, 89, 103, 112–13, 114–15, 178, 194n9
Shibutani, Shinya, 128
Shope, Richard, 150
Silbart, Lawrence, 184n4
Silent Spring (Carson), 87
simplification and oversimplification, 27
Skakkebaek, Niels, 89, 103. See also "Evidence for Decreasing Quality of Semen During the Past 50 Years"
Slovic, Paul, 42–43
smallpox, 167
smokeless tobacco, 11
smoking: dose-response relationship, 103; increased lung cancer risk, 14, 15–16, 26; magnitude of exposure, 15, 38; public perception of threat, 43, 179
society: health discourse embedded in, 32–34, 33; Latour's "hybrid" concept and, 35, 110; and the scientific establishment, xvii, 5, 32–34, 33, 175–76. See also public, the
specific absorption rate (SAR), 63
sperm. See semen quality
statistics, assessing findings through, 22–23

stomach cancer, 29, 56. See also H. pylori
"Strong Inference" (Platt), 30–31
study design, 26, 27, 63–66, 105–6, 113
Sumpter, John, 114
sun exposure, 43, 179
Sunstein, Cass, 53–55, 84, 189n25

Taiwan, 136–38
Teeguarden, Justin, 103, 106–7
testicular cancer, 85–86, 89, 98, 100–101
testicular dysgenesis syndrome (TDS), 89, 98–101, 112, 196n37. See also semen quality
Thinking, Fast and Slow (Kahneman), 51–53
thinking outside the box, 2–3
tobacco, smokeless, 11. See also smoking
Tolstoy, Leo, 57
toxicology, 103–4, 122
translational research, 121
trebuchet-siege cartoon, 41–42, 42
Tversky, Amos, 51, 52. See also Kahneman, Daniel

Uganda, 144–45, 147, 166. See also Burkitt's lymphoma
ulcers (stomach), 29, 49, 56
United Nations, 47
urothelial cancer, 118, 120, 125, 129, 131–40. See also Chinese herbs nephropathy; Balkan endemic nephropathy

vaccines: fraudulent study linking autism to, 11, 45, 185n3; HPV vaccines, 7, 56, 161–62, 165–67; mistrust of, 11, 165; not a threat, 177
Vanherweghem, Jean-Louis, 116–17, 118, 119
viruses, and cancer, 144–49, 180, 203n11. See also Burkitt's lymphoma; cervical cancer
Vogelstein, Bert, 133, 135

Volkow, Nora, 79–80
vom Saal, Frederick, 102, 103, 105–6

Wakefield, Andrew, 45, 185n3
Wald, Abraham, 2–3, 29, 184n4
Warren, Robin, 29
WHO. *See* World Health Organization
"Why Most Published Research Findings are False" (Ioannidis), 22–23. *See also* Ioannidis, John P.
Wilcox, Allen, 111–12
wildlife, synthetic chemicals and, 86, 88–89, 91, 94
Wingspread statement, 88–89

wireless telecommunications, 62. *See also* cell phones and brain cancer
World Cancer Research Fund/American Institute for Cancer Research, 21
World Health Organization (WHO), 9, 108, 125, 167
World War II aerial bombing campaign, 1–3

X-rays, 59, 62, 62. *See also* radiation

Zoeller, Thomas, 103
zur Hausen, Harald, 29, 148–52, 161, 167, 180